普通高等教育"十一五"国家级规划教材

全国高等医药院校药学类专业第二轮实验双语教材

生药学实验与指导

（第 2 版）

主　　编　李会军

副主编　高　雯　黄　芸　付　钰

编　　者　（以姓氏笔画为序）

付　钰（河南中医药大学）

年四辉（皖南医学院）

毕志明（中国药科大学）

李会军（中国药科大学）

陆　续（中国药科大学）

陈　君（中国药科大学）

高　雯（中国药科大学）

黄　芸（河北医科大学）

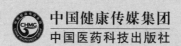中国健康传媒集团

中国医药科技出版社

内容提要

本教材为"全国高等医药院校药学类专业第二轮实验双语教材"之一，为中英文对照实验类教材。全书共三篇三十七个实验，内容包括基础性实验、验证性实验和设计性与综合性实验。本教材供全国医药院校本科、专科的实验教学使用，也可作为相关专业的继续教育教材或自学教材的参考书。

图书在版编目（CIP）数据

生药学实验与指导：汉英对照 / 李会军主编 . —2 版 . —北京：中国医药科技出版社，2022.8

普通高等教育"十一五"国家级规划教材　全国高等医药院校药学类专业第二轮实验双语教材

ISBN 978 - 7 - 5214 - 3286 - 2

Ⅰ . ①生… Ⅱ . ①李… Ⅲ . ①生药学 - 实验 - 双语教学 - 高等学校 - 教材 - 汉、英　Ⅳ . ①R93 - 33

中国版本图书馆 CIP 数据核字（2022）第 121340 号

美术编辑　陈君杞

版式设计　南博文化

出版　**中国健康传媒集团** | 中国医药科技出版社

地址　北京市海淀区文慧园北路甲 22 号

邮编　100082

电话　发行：010 - 62227427　邮购：010 - 62236938

网址　www. cmstp. com

规格　889 × 1194mm $\frac{1}{16}$

印张　11 $\frac{1}{2}$

彩插　12

字数　321 千字

初版　2007 年 2 月第 1 版

版次　2022 年 8 月第 2 版

印次　2022 年 8 月第 1 次印刷

印刷　三河市万龙印装有限公司

经销　全国各地新华书店

书号　ISBN 978 - 7 - 5214 - 3286 - 2

定价　**39.00 元**

版权所有　盗版必究

举报电话：010 - 62228771

本社图书如存在印装质量问题请与本社联系调换

获取新书信息、投稿、为图书纠错，请扫码联系我们。

教学是学校人才培养的中心环节，实验教学是这一环节的重要组成部分。"全国高等医药院校药学类专业第二轮实验双语教材"是中国药科大学自 2005 年以来坚持药学实践教学改革，突出提高学生动手能力、创新思维，通过承担教育部"世行贷款——21 世纪初高等教育教学改革项目"等多项教改课题，逐步建设完善的一套与药学各专业学科理论课程紧密结合的高水平双语实验教材。

本轮修订，适逢"全国高等医药院校药学类专业第五轮规划教材"及 2020 年版《中国药典》出版，本教材的修订突出与新版理论教材知识的结合，对接 2020 年版《中国药典》、新版《药品质量管理规范》（GMP）等新颁布法典法规；为更好地服务于新时期高等院校药学教育与人才培养的需要，在上一版的基础上，进一步体现了各门实验课程自身独立性、系统性和科学性，又充分考虑到各门实验课程之间的联系与衔接。本教材具有以下特点。

1. 适应医药行业对人才的要求，体现行业特色　契合新时期药学人才需求的变化，使修订后的教材符合 2020 年版《中国药典》及新版 GMP、新版 GSP 等国家标准、法规和规范以及新版国家执业药师资格考试大纲等行业最新要求。

2. 更新完善内容，打造教材精品　在上版教材基础上进一步优化、精炼和充实内容。紧密结合"全国高等医药院校药学类专业第五轮规划教材"，强调与实际需求相结合，进一步提高教材质量。

3. 坚持双语体系，强调素质培养　教材以实践教学为突破口，采用双语体系编写，有利于加快药学教育国际接轨，提高学生的科技英语水平，进一步提升学生整体素质。

"全国高等医药院校药学类专业第二轮实验双语教材"历经十五年四次建设，在各个时期广大编写教师的努力下，在广大使用教材师生的支持下日臻完善。本轮教材的出版，必将对推动新时期我国高等药学教育的发展产生积极而深远的影响。希望广大师生在教学实践中对本套教材提出宝贵意见，以便今后进一步修订完善，共同打造精品教材。

吴晓明

全国高等医药院校药学类专业第五轮规划教材常务编委会主任委员

2019 年 10 月

前言
Preface

生药学是一门实践性很强的学科。《生药学实验与指导》是《生药学》（第4版）的配套教材。本书以生药学课程教学大纲规定的实验内容为主，并做了必要的补充与扩展，使学生通过实践，除了能够牢固掌握生药学的基本概念、基本理论和基本实验技能外，还同时具备解决复杂性、系统性问题的研究创新能力。

本书分为三篇。第一篇为"基础性实验"，主要包括生药性状与显微鉴别方法、生药薄层色谱鉴别方法、生药水分、灰分、挥发油、浸出物、重金属及有害元素、残留农药等限量检查方法等。第二篇为"验证性实验"，共有33个代表性生药，实验内容主要包括生药性状鉴别、显微鉴别、理化鉴别等内容。第三篇为"设计性与综合性实验"，主要包括混合生药粉末鉴别、生药DNA分子鉴别、生药指纹图谱与特征图谱鉴别、生药多成分含量测定、生药质量标准研究与制订。此外，为了便于学生参考和查询，在书后附录还收录有生药鉴定常见专业词汇。

本书为全国医药院校本科、专科的实验教学用书，也可作为相关专业的继续教育用教材或自学教材的参考书。使用时，各院校可根据自身的人才培养目标，并结合实验教学条件，选择适当的实验项目开展实验教学活动。

本教材的编写得到中国药科大学生药学课程教学团队的大力支持。中国药科大学生药学专业研究生王俏蕾、钱朵朵、孟欢欢、邱芳宁、李富贵等协助主编做了部分文字、图片校对工作，在此一并致以深深的谢意。

限于时间和水平，教材中难免存在许多不足，敬请各位同仁提出宝贵意见，以便今后修订。

编者
2022 年 5 月

第一篇　基础性实验

Chapter 1　Basic Experiments

实验一　生药的性状鉴别

【实验目的】

1. 掌握生药的性状鉴别方法。
2. 掌握常用的性状鉴别术语。

【实验指导】

1. 性状鉴别的内容

性状鉴别主要是采用眼看、手摸、鼻闻、口尝、水试、火试等简便的方法鉴别中药材的真伪。性状鉴别的内容包括形状、大小、颜色、表面特征、质地、折断面的特征、气味、水试、火试等。

2. 观察结果的描述

（1）形状　药材的形状与药用部位有关，每种药材的形状一般比较固定，是鉴别真伪的重要依据之一。如根类药材有圆形、圆锥形、纺锤形等；皮类药材有卷筒状、板片状等；种子类药材有圆球形、扁圆柱形等。可借鉴老药工对药材的经验鉴别术语进行描述，如马头蛇尾瓦楞身等。

（2）大小　药材的大小指长短、粗细、厚薄。要得出比较正确的大小数值，应观察较多的样品。如测量的大小与规定有差异时，可允许有少量高于或低于规定的数值。很小的种子类药材则应在放大镜下测量。也可放在 1mm 方格的纸上，每 10 粒紧密排成一行，测量后求其平均值。

（3）颜色　各种药材的颜色不尽相同。药材若加工或贮藏不当，其固有色泽就会改变，这也预示着质量发生变化。当药材具有复合色调时，应以后一种色调为主，如黄棕色以棕色为主。观察时一般在日光下进行。

（4）表面特征　药材表面光滑或粗糙，有无皱纹、皮孔、毛绒等。双子叶植物的根类药材顶部有的带有根茎；单子叶植物有的具膜质鳞皮；蕨类植物的根茎常常带有叶柄残基和鳞片。皮类药材表面含有地衣斑和皮孔；叶类药材有的有毛茸。这些特征的有无和存在的情况常是鉴别药材的重要依据，应仔细观察。

（5）质地　是指药材的软硬、坚韧、疏松、致密、黏性或粉性等特征。有些药材因加工方法不同，质地也不同。如盐附子易吸潮变软，黑顺片则质硬而脆；含淀粉多的药材经蒸煮加工，则因淀粉糊化，干燥后而质地坚实，如白芍。在经验鉴别中，有很多用于形容

1

药材质地的术语，如"松泡"（南沙参）、"粉性"（贝母）、"油润"（当归）、"角质"（郁金）、"柴性"（黄柏）等。

（6）折断面　药材折断时的现象，如易折断或不易折断，有无粉尘散落及折断时的断面特征。自然折断的断面应注意是平坦，还是显纤维性、颗粒性或裂片状，断面有无胶丝等。用刀片切成横切面，以便观察皮部与木部的比例、维管束的排列形状、射线的分布及异型构造等。

（7）气味　药材独特的气与味，直接以鼻闻和口尝进行鉴别。含挥发性物质的药材，大多有特殊的香气，如肉桂、薄荷、丁香等。气不明显的药材可切碎后用热水浸泡一下再闻。若药材味道发生改变，就可考虑其品种和质量问题。注意剧毒药不宜口尝，毒性较小的生药口尝时也要小心，取量要少。

（8）水试　利用某些药材在水中的特殊现象来鉴别药材，如秦皮水浸液具碧蓝色荧光；车前子水浸泡，体积膨胀；牛黄的水浸液染指甲而俗称为"挂甲"。

（9）火试　利用某些药材火烧时，产生特殊的气味、颜色、烟雾、响声等来鉴别药材。如麝香灼烧时，香气浓烈，无臭气，灰烬白色；血竭粉末置于滤纸上灼烧时，对光透视显血红色，无扩散的油斑，无残留的灰烬；乳香、没药火试冒浓烟，有香气等。

【仪器与试剂】

1. 仪器
毫米刻度尺、手持式放大镜、培养皿、烧杯、酒精灯等。

2. 试剂
蒸馏水等。

【实验材料】

黄芪（药材及饮片）、海马、防风、三七、党参、川贝母（松贝、青贝及炉贝）、天麻（春麻及冬麻）、秦皮、海金沙。

【实验步骤】

1. 性状观察与测量
观察黄芪的外观形状，测量其长度、厚度、直径，观察表面特征和颜色、断面特征和颜色，嗅气，尝味。

2. 经验鉴别
对照老药工总结的经验鉴别术语，观察海马、防风、三七、党参、川贝母（松贝、青贝及炉贝）、天麻（春麻及冬麻）的外形特征。

3. 水试
取秦皮 3~5g 置烧杯中，加水 25ml，浸泡约 10 分钟，在日光下观察浸出液颜色。

4. 火试
取海金沙少量，撒于酒精灯火焰上方，观察现象。

【实验报告】

1. 记录对黄芪的观察或测量结果，注意描述的先后顺序。

2. 记录水试秦皮、火试海金沙的结果。

【思考题】

性状鉴别方法的主要适用对象是哪些生药？该鉴别方法有何优缺点？

Experiment 1　Macroscopical Identification of Crude Drugs

【Objective】

1. To master the macroscopical identification method of crude drugs.
2. To master the commonly used characteristic terms for identification of crude drugs.

【Principle】

1. Macroscopical identification method

Macroscopical identification of crude drug is mainly based on the characters acquired by human senses such as seeing, touching, smelling, tasting. Usually, the identification characters include shape, size, color, external, texture, fracture, odour, and taste. In some cases, the characts observed from water – based test and fire – based test are equally important.

2. Description of the identification characters

(1)Shape:The shape of crude drug varies with the medicinally used parts. For example, the roots are often round, conical, spindle – shaped, and so on. The barks are roll, slab, etc. The seeds are spherical, flat cylindrical. In this respect, many useful identification terms are summarized by sophisticated pharmacists.

(2)Size:The size of crude drug refers to the length and the thickness. To obtain more accurate values, large – scale samples should be observed. If there is a difference between the measured values and the specified, a small amount of samples with higher or lower values than the specified can be allowed. The very fine seeds should be measured under a magnifying glass. It can also be placed on a 1mm square paper, and every ten seeds are arranged in a row tightly. Then the average value is calculated after measurement.

(3)Color:The colors of various crude drugs are different. If the crude drugs are improperly processed or stored, their inherent colors will change, indicating the possibility of quality change. When a crude drug exhibits a kind of composite color, the main color should be postpositionally described. For instance, in the composite color of yellow – brown, brown is the primary color. Observation is generally carried out in sunlight.

(4)External:The external of crude drug might be smooth or rough, with or without wrinkles, lenticels, and trichomes, and so on. Some roots of dicotyledons plants have rhizomes on the top, some roots of monocotyledonous plants have membranous scales, while the rhizomes of ferns often have petiole residues and scales. Usually, barks show lichen spots and lenticels on the surface, leaves have trichomes. The presence and absence of these identification characters are very important and deserve careful observistion.

(5) Texture: It refers to the characters of softness, toughness, looseness, compactness, stickiness or powderiness of crude drugs. Crude drugs have different textures due to the different processing methods. For example, salted aconite root is easy to absorb moisture and become soft, while Heishun Pian is hard and brittle. If the starch – rich crude drug, such as Radix Paeoniae Alba, is processed by steaming, it will become gelatinized with a solid texture. There are many empirical terms to describe the texture of the crude drugs, such as "spongy" (Adenophorae Radix), "starchy" (Fritillariae Bulbus), "oily" (Angelicae Sinensis Radix), "horny" (Curcumae Radix), "woody" (Phellodendri Chinensis Cortex), and so on.

(6) Fracture: It refers to the characters when the crude drugs are broken, such as easily or not easily broken, whether there is dust scattered. The fracture that is naturally broken might show flat, fibrous, granular or splintery. Attention should be paid to the presence or absence of glue threads on the section. The following characters including the ratio of bark to wood, the arranging shape of vascular bundles, the distribution of rays, or the abnormal structure, can be observedin the cutting fracture.

(7) Odour and taste: The unique odour and taste of a crude drug is determined by smelling and tasting. Most of the crude drugs containing volatile substances have a special aroma, such as Cinnamomi Cortex, Menthae Haplocalycis Herba, and Caryophylli Flos. Crude drugs with no obvious odour can be chopped and soaked in hot water before smelling. If the taste of a crude drug changes, its quality may also change. Notably, the hypertoxic crude drugs should not be tasted, and the less toxic crude drugs should be tasted carefully with a small amount.

(8) Water – based test: The special phenomena when soaking in water can be used to identify crude drugs. For instance, the aqueous solution by soaking Fraxini Cortex shows light blue fluorescence; Plantaginis Semenwill dramatically swell when immersed in water. As respect to Bovis Calculus, its soaking solution can stain nails into to yellow, commonly known as "Guajia".

(9) Fire – based test: The special phenomena when burning can be used to identify crude drugs, including odour, color, smoke, noise, etc. For instance, aromatic odour can be smelt and white ash is residued when Moschus is burnt. When the powder of Draconis Sanguis is placed on the filter paper and burned, it presents bright red and shows no spreading oil stains, and residual ashes are invisible. When burning Olibanum and Myrrha, it shows an oily look with blach smoke and aromatic odour.

【Instruments and Reagents】

1. Instruments
Millimeter scale, hand – held magnifying glass, petri dish, alcohol lamp, beaker.
2. Reagents
Distilled water.

【Materials】

Astragali Radix (including crude drug and decoction pieces), Hippocampus, Saposhnikoviae Radix, Notoginseng Radix et Rhizoma, Codonopsis Radix, Fritillariae Cirrhosae Bulbus (including Song bei, Qing bei and Lu bei), Gastrodiae Rhizome (including Chunma and Dongma), Fraxini Cortex, Lygodii Spora.

【Experimental Procedures】

1. Observation and description of identification characters

Observe the appearance and shape of Astragali Radix, measure the length, thickness, diameter. Observe the color and charaters in surface and fracture views, respectively. Smell and taste.

2. Empirical identification

According to the empirical identification terms summarized by the sophisticated pharmacists, observe the appearance characters of Hippocampus, Saposhnikoviae Radix, Notoginseng Radix et Rhizoma, Codonopsis Radix, Fritillariae Cirrhosae Bulbus, and Gastrodiae Rhizome.

3. Water – based test

Weighabout 3 – 5g of Fraxini Cortex to a beaker. Add 25ml of water, macerate for about 10min. Then observe the color of solution under sunlight.

4. Fire – based test

Take a small amount of Lygodii Spora and sprinkle on the flame of the alcohol lamp, observe the phenomena.

【Assignments】

1. Record the observation and the measurement results of Astragali Radix.

2. Record the phenomenaby the water – based test of Fraxini Cortex and the fire – based test of Lygodii Spora.

【Discussion】

Which kind of crude drugs are applicable to the macroscopical identification method? What are the advantages and disadvantages of this identification method?

实验二　生药显微标本片的制作与显微镜的使用

【实验目的】

1. 掌握生药显微鉴别的基本制片技术。
2. 了解显微镜的构造，掌握显微镜的使用方法。

【实验指导】

1. 生药显微标本片的制作

在生药的显微鉴定工作中，首先须将样品制成显微标本片，然后才能在显微镜下观察。根据鉴别对象和目的不同，生药显微标本片的制作方法有徒手制片法、粉末制片法、表面制片法、石蜡制片法等。

（1）徒手制片法　是利用剃刀或保险刀片把新鲜的、预先固定好的或软化的材料切成薄片，不染色或经简单染色，用水封片后观察。徒手制片一般供临时观察用。

（2）粉末制片法　是粉末状生药、以生药粉末入药的中成药的显微鉴定的标本片的制片方法。一般药材经过粉碎、过筛后制片，特别坚硬的药材可用锉刀将其搓成粉末。粉末制片法主要用于观察细胞和细胞后含物的形态特征。

（3）表面制片法　适用于观察叶类、花类生药以及浆果、草质茎、根茎等的表皮显微特征，便于观察表皮细胞的形态、气孔的类型、毛绒的特征及着生情况等。

（4）石蜡制片法　是利用石蜡能渗透到材料组织内部的特性，作为材料的填充剂和包埋剂，用旋转切片机进行切片的方法。此法可切得厚仅 $4 \sim 5\mu m$ 的薄片，因此可以清晰地观察药材组织结构，且可永久保存，但步骤较多，操作费时。

2. 显微镜的构造

显微镜主要由装置光学系统的机械部分与保证成像的光学部分组成，如图 2 - 1。

（1）机械部分主要包括镜座、镜臂、镜筒、载物台、物镜转换器、焦距调节装置等。

①镜座用于保持显微镜的稳定与平衡。

②镜臂用于支持镜筒及取放显微镜时握持之用。

③镜筒为一中空的金属圆筒，用以固定物镜与目镜间的距离。以双筒倾斜式为常见。镜筒中转折处装有棱镜，使光线转折45°。

④载物台用于放置载玻片（可由夹压片固定），中央有一通光孔。装置较完善的显微镜，载物台一侧附有移动杆，可控制载玻片前后左右的移动。利用移动器上的游标尺可观察、记录被检品的位置，便于再观察或重新拍照。

⑤物镜转换盘具有 3～6 个螺旋口，每个螺旋口配置有不同放大倍率的物镜。通过转动转换盘，可利用不同放大倍率的物镜。

⑥焦距调节装置通过控制镜筒与载物台的升降，调节物镜与标本间的距离。主要包括粗调节器和细调节器 2 个部分。外端一般是粗调节器，内段一般是细调节器。

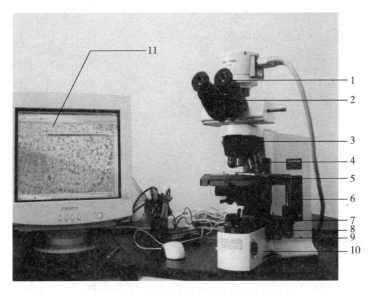

图 2 - 1　光学显微镜的构造示意图

Figure 2 - 1　The structure of the optical microscope

1. 目镜（eyepieces）；2. 镜筒（draw - tube）；3. 物镜转换盘（substage condenser）；4. 物镜（objective）

5. 载物台（stage）；6. 载物台移动杆（shift lever of stage）；7. 聚光器（condenser adjustment）；

8. 细调焦螺旋（fine - focusing knob）；9. 粗调焦螺旋（coarse - focusing knob）；

10. 镜座（base）；11. 数字显示器（digital displayer）

（2）光学部分主要由一系列放大透镜组合而成。除了主要用于放大的透镜组外，尚有光密度调节装置、滤光片、光源等。

①物镜是决定显微镜性能的最重要部分，内装有多组复式透镜。镜筒长，透镜组数多，放大率则大。一般放大率在 10 倍以下者，被称为"低倍物镜"；放大率在 40 倍以上者，被称为"高倍物镜"。为防止散射、漫射，在物镜与标本间选用香柏油或特别浸润油作为介质进行观察时，被称为"油镜"，放大率一般在 100 倍。

②目镜内装有一组放大率较小的透镜组，其作用在于将物镜所成图像进一步放大。就分辨力而言，目镜不能提高图像的质量。目镜表面都刻有放大率，如 5 ×，10 ×，15 × 等三种。

③光密度调节装置：聚光器由数片透镜组成，位于载物台下方，用于将光线集中到所要观察的标本上。聚光器的一侧，尚装有升降调节轮，供汇聚光线密度所用。通常刻在上方透镜边框上的数字是代表最大的数值孔径。在低倍镜观察时，可将最上面的一块上透镜移除光路之外，使得聚光镜的数值孔径变小。通过调节可变光阑的开放程度，从而得到透镜边框上的数字所代表的不同数值孔径，更好地发挥显微镜的观察效果。一般说来，光阑孔径开大，光量度会加强，但又会降低物镜的解像力。因此，聚光器的光阑开孔最好为物镜数值孔径的 60% ~70%。

场光阑位于光源的上方，主要功能是靠减少物镜反射光斑来控制图像的光。一般在明视野时，可将场光阑全部打开，直到在显微镜中可以看到它的整个圆形视野为止。

【仪器与试剂】

1. 仪器

显微镜、刀片、镊子、解剖针、酒精灯、吸水纸等。

2. 试剂

乙醇、水合氯醛、稀甘油、蒸馏水等。

【实验材料】

麦冬、山药、大青叶（新鲜叶片或干燥药材）。

【实验步骤】

1. 生药显微标本片的制作

（1）徒手制片法　一般是先将材料切成 2~3cm 的小段，坚硬的材料可用水煮、50% 乙醇–甘油（1∶1）浸泡，软化后再切片。若材料过软时，则可置 70%~95% 乙醇中浸泡 20~30 分钟。切片时，左手拇指和食指夹住材料，用中指托起，材料要高于手指。将刀口放在外缘的 1/4 左右处，刀片贴切面平拉，不要担心切片太薄或不完整而将刀口向下。注意切忌来回拉锯。将切下的薄片用湿毛笔转移到盛水的培养皿中，再选最薄的切片放在载玻片上观察，也可用 0.1% 番红溶液将细胞核及木质化、栓质化的细胞壁染色后再观察。

取麦冬药材，采用徒手制片法制作显微标本片 3 张。

（2）粉末制片法　一般是先将药材烘干、粉碎，过 5~6 号筛。取粉末适量（约半粒大米粒大小），加水（不透化，观察淀粉粒），或加水合氯醛，加热、透化，再加稀甘油（观察细胞、草酸钙结晶等后含物），或加乙醇（观察橙皮苷或菊糖团块）。

取山药药材，采用粉末制片法制作显微标本片 3 张。

（3）表面制片法　较薄的材料可整体封藏，其他材料可撕取或削取表皮制作。若为干的材料，如较薄的叶、花类生药可用冷水浸泡至能伸展、恢复原样后，用刀片在表面轻轻浅划一刀，用小镊子从切口处撕取表皮。若为较软的浆果类，可直接削取表皮。如较硬的则需要经软化处理。水合氯醛试液透化后，加甘油封藏。

取大青叶（干燥药材或新鲜叶片），采用表面制片法制作显微标本片 3 张。

2. 显微镜的使用方法

使用显微镜时，应注意"两先两后"：即先低倍，后高倍；先粗调，后微调。操作时，应徐徐将物镜下降，以至几乎接近盖玻片，然后再徐徐提升，调整合适的焦距。应先用低倍镜对标本片进行全面观察；如再对某一特定的部分作进一步较详细的观察时，则必须先把该部分移至视野中心，再换用高倍镜进行观察。由于物体本身具有一定的厚度与不同的透明度，故观察过程中，尚需不断轻微调节细调节器。同时应按照物体透明度的大小，将聚光器或虹彩光圈作适当的调节，以便对物体的结构获得清晰、完整的概貌。

观察完毕后，必须把物镜转离光路，取下标本片，使显微镜恢复至非工作状态放回原处。

【实验报告】

1. 简要记录徒手制片法、粉末制片法、表面制片法的操作步骤。
2. 提交各种合格制片各一张。

【思考题】

1. 使用显微镜要注意哪些事项？
2. 如何才能制备出合格的显微标本片？

Experiment 2　Preparation of Microscopical Specimen Slides of Crude Drugs and Usage of Microscope

【Objective】

1. To master the preparation techniques of microscopical specimen slides of crude drugs.

2. To know the structure of a microscope and masater its proper using method.

【Principle】

1. Preparation of microscopical specimen slides of crude drugs

Making aqualified specimen slide is a prerequisite to microscopical identification. There are four preparation methods, viz. freehand slicing method, powder slicing method, surface slicing method and paraffin slicing method.

（1）Freeh and slicing method：The fresh or pre – soften materials are sliced into thin slices with razor blade, and mounted with water. The prepared slides are usually non – staining or simply staining, suitable for temporary observation.

（2）Powder slicing method：The crude drugs or Chinese patent drugs containing powdered crude drugs are pulverized and sieved, then mounted. The prepared slides are mainly suitable for observation of cells and cell ergastic substances.

（3）Surface slicing method：The method is suitable for observation of epidermal tissues from leaves, fruits or herbaceous stems. The observation points include the morphology of epidermal cells, stomata type, and epidermal trichomes.

（4）Paraffin slicing method：The fresh or pre – soften materials are sliced into thin slices with rotary microtome, using paraffin as stuffing agent and embedding medium. The slices are $4 - 5 \mu m$ in thickness, ensuring anatomy structures of objects being clearly observed. The prepared slides can be stored permanently, although the preparation procedures are tedious and time – consuming.

2. Structure of microscope

Typically, a microscope is mainly composed of two parts：the mechanical system and the optical system.

（1）Mechanical system：including the base, the arm, the draw – tube, the stage, the nosepiece, and the focusing knob, etc. .

①Base：A unit supports the microscope and keeps it steady.

② Arm：An arm supports the draw – tube and can be used as the handle.

③Draw – tube：A hollow metal chamber is used to fix the distance between the objective lens and the eyepiece.

④ Stage：A platform is used to place and fix the slide. There is a hole in the center, through which light can pass. A well – equipped microscope has a shift lever, which controls the movement direction of the slide.

⑤Substage condenser：A disc has 3 – 6 screw poles. Each of them is fitted with objective lenses of difference magnifications.

⑥Focusing knob：A device is used to adjust the distance between objective lense and specimen by raising and lowering the draw – tube and stage. It mainly includes the coarse – focusing knob and fine – focusing knob. Generally, the outer one is a coarse regulator, and the inner is a fine regulator.

（2）Optical system：including a set of magnifying lenses, the light density control, the light filter, and the light source etc.

①Objective：They are very important to the function of a microscope, and there are several sets of compound lenses inside. Longer draw – tube and more sets of lenses result in higher magnifying power. Generally, the lower powder objective lens is below 10 magnifications and the high powder objective lens is above 40 magnifications. In order to prevent scattering and diffusing, add cedar oil or other special oils between the objective lenses and the specimen, and the objective lens can be 100 magnifications, also called "oil immersion".

②Eyepiece：They contain a set of lenses in lower magnifying power. It can further magnify the image produced by the objective lenses, but cannot promote the quality of the image. Magnifications are carved on the surface of the eyepiece, such as $5 \times, 10 \times, 15 \times$.

③Light density control

Condenser adjustment：It is composed of several lenses and located below the stage. It is used to concentrate light on the inspected specimen. This is an adjust knob on the side of microscope which can lift or lower the condenser to change the light density. The numbers usually engraved on the upper lenses frame represent the largest numerical aperture. When observing with a low magnification lens, the uppermost lens can be removed from the optical path to make the numerical aperture of the condenser smaller. By adjusting the opening degree of the iris diaphragm, the different numerical apertures represented by the numbers on the lens frame can be obtained, and the observation effect of the microscope can be better exerted. If the iris diaphragm aperture is increased, the light quantity will be strengthened, but it will reduce the resolution of the objective lens. Therefore, the aperture of the condenser is preferably $60\% \sim 70\%$ of the numerical aperture of the objective lens.

Iris diaphragm：It is located above the light source, and used to control the image light by reducing the light reflected from the objective lens. In the bright field, the iris diaphragm can be fully opened until the entire circular field can be seen in the microscope.

【Instruments and Reagents】

1. Instruments

Microscope, one – side blade, nippers, dissecting needle, alcohol lamp, blotting paper.

2. Reagents

Dilute glycerin, chloral hydratetest solution.

【Materials】

Ophiopogonis Radix, Dioscoreae Rhizoma, Isatidis Folium(fresh leaves or dried crude drug).

【Experimental Procedures】

1. Preparation of microscopical specimen slides

(1)Freehand slicing method：Generally, the material is cutted into small pecies with length of 2 ~ 3cm. For those harder materials, softening treatments including boiling in water, or soaking with amixture of 50% ethanol and glycerin(1:1) are needed. For those relatively softer materials, soaking with 70% ~95% ethanol for 20 ~ 30min is recommended. When cutting, clamp the material with thumb and forefinger, upbear with middle finger so as tomake the material higher than fingers. Put the blade on the 1/4 portion of outer margin, move the blade in a flatwise orientation to obtain slices. Notably, do not cut the material in a downward direction! Additionally, never move the blade back and forth. Transfer the cut slices to a culture dish containing water with writing brush. Choose the thinnest slice, and put it on a glass slide for observation. Staining with with 0.1% safranine solution is used for observation of cell nucleus, lignified and suberized cell walls.

Prepare 3 pieces of microscopical specimen slides of Ophiopogonis Radix, by the above described method.

(2)Powder slicing method：Firstly, the material is dried and pulverized, sieved through No. 5 –6 sieve. Then, disperse a very small quantity of the powdered crude drug on a glass slide, add 2 – 3 drops of water for observation of starch grains, or add chloral hydrate and maintain gentle boiling for a short time, followed by adding dilute glycerin for observation of cells and their ergastic substances like calcium oxalate crystals, or add ethanol for observation of hesperidin or inulin.

Prepare 3 pieces of microscopical specimen slides of Dioscoreae Rhizoma, by the above described method.

(3)Surface slicing method：For those thick materials, the whole body can be directly mounted; for other materials, epidermal parts should be peeled off for mounting. For the dried materials, like thick leaves or flowers, soaking in cold water until unfolded is nessary. Then make a light cut on the surface with blade, take a piece of epidermal parts from the cut. For a soft berry, the epidermal part can be easily peeled off. As respect to the hard berries, softening treatments are needed. Permeabilize with chloral hydrate and mount with glycerin.

Prepare 3 pieces of microscopical specimen slides of Isatidis Folium, by the above described method.

2. Observation under a microscope

There are two sequence rules for using a microscope：one rule is that the observing sequence is from low power objective to high power objective, the other is that adjusting sequence is from coarse – focusing knob to fine – focusing knob. Generally, the first step is lowering the objective lens carefully until very approaching to the cover glass. Then lift slowly and look for the target at the same time. Prelimilarily observe under lower power objective to examine the material totally, subsequently move the image from specified portion observe to the central field of view, observeunder high power objective. Finnaly, adjust the focusing knobs(from coarse to fine)so as to clearly imaging. Due to the thickness and transparency of the specimen, fine knob should be adjusted slightly during the observation. Also, the condenser can be adjusted according to the transparency of the specimen in order to showa clear and integrated structure of the specimen.

When the observation is completed, it is sure to turn objective away from the light path, take off the specimen slide, restore the microscope to its initial state.

【Assignments】

1. Describe the experimental procedure for preparing microscopical specimen slides with different methods.

2. Show the qualified microscopical specimen slides.

【Discussion】

1. What are the matters needing attention during using a microscope?

2. How to prepare a qualified microscopical specimen slide?

实验三　生药显微测量与显微描绘

【实验目的】

1. 掌握显微测量和显微描绘方法。

【实验指导】

1. 显微测量标尺

在生药的显微鉴别工作中，经常要用显微测量标尺测量所观察的微细目标物的大小。测量长度的显微量尺有目镜量尺和载台量尺两种。此外，还有一种网格式标尺，可用来计算数目和测量面积。

目镜量尺是置于目镜内的、在一块直径 18 ～20mm 的圆形玻璃片上刻有精细刻度的标尺（图 3 – 1）。刻度全长 1cm 或 0.5cm，精确等分为 50 ～200 小格。

载台量尺是一种在载玻片中央刻有微细刻度的特制标尺（图 3 – 2）。刻度全长 1mm，精确等分为 10 大格，100 小格，故每小格 10μm。刻度外围有一小黑圈，以便易于找到标尺。

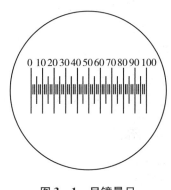

图 3 – 1　目镜量尺

Figure 3 – 1　Measuring scale of eyepieces

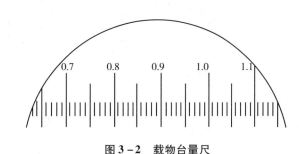

图 3 – 2　载物台量尺

Figure 3 – 2　Measuring scale of stage

2. 显微绘图法

生药的组织特征图可分为组织简图和组织详图两大类。

（1）组织简图，一般不画出细胞的形状，而是用不同的符号代表不同的组织特征。一般通用的特征符号见图 3 – 3。

（2）组织详图用来表述生药组织中各种细胞及后含物的形状及排列情况。在组织详图中，每个细胞的形状、壁厚、纹孔、层纹等特征，都要尽可能画准确。

生药的显微绘图有徒手绘图法、显微描绘器绘图法等。随着技术的发展，数码显微摄影装置能实时、高保真采集显微镜下的图像，在生药显微鉴定中的应用也日益普及。

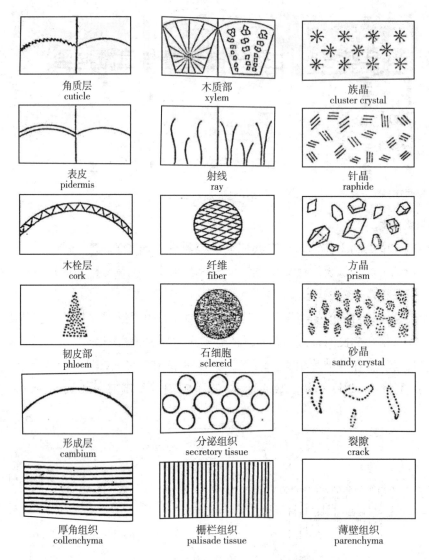

图 3 - 3　显微组织简图常用代表符号图

Figure 3 - 3　Reprenting symbols of microstructures

【仪器与试剂】

目镜量尺（精确等分为 100 小格）、载台量尺（1mm 长，精确等分为 100 小格，每小格长为 0.01mm，即 $10\mu m$）、描绘目镜等。

【实验材料】

甘草横切面永久制片。

【实验步骤】

1. 目镜量尺的标化

目镜量尺所代表的长度是随所使用的显微镜的镜筒长度、目镜和物镜的放大倍率而改变的，因此在测定前必须对在即将采用的光学组合系统下目镜量尺每小格所代表的长度进行标化。标化时，将载台量尺置于显微镜的载台上，将目镜量尺放入目镜筒内。将载台量尺刻度移至视野中央，调焦至刻度清晰，然后转动目镜，让两种量尺的刻度平行，再移动载台量尺使两种量尺左端"0"刻度重合，再向右找出第二条重合线，根据两条重合线间两种量尺的小格数，按下式计算出目镜量尺每小格所代表的实际长度（图3－4）。

$$目镜量尺每小格所代表实际长度（\mu m） = \frac{两条重合线间载台量尺的小格数 \times 10}{两条重合线间目镜量尺的小格数}$$

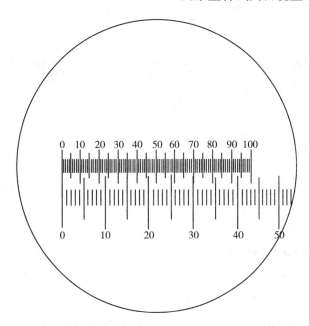

图 3－4 表示视野中目镜测量尺与载物台量尺的重合线

Figure 3－4 The concidence line between the eyepieces measuring scale and the stage measuring scale

分别在低倍镜及高倍镜下标化目镜量尺，并计算目镜量尺每一小格相当的微米数。

2. 显微测量

以甘草横切面标本片代替载台量尺放置于载物台上，用已标化好的目镜量尺测量目标物的大小（如木质部导管的直径）。

3. 显微描绘

取甘草根横切片先在低倍镜下观察，从外向内观察其构造的各部位，再在高倍镜下重点观察韧皮部、形成层及木质部区域，选择组织细胞完整、轮廓清晰、有代表性的组织细胞进行描绘。

（1）徒手绘图法直接用铅笔对显微镜中观察到的物象作图。可一边观察一边绘图，反复对照修改，直至满意。

（2）显微描绘器绘图法将描绘器安放在显微镜镜筒上，描绘时注意调节显微镜的焦距，并调节光亮使显微镜视野中及描绘纸上的光线强弱相当，视野中的物像和绘图用的铅笔尖像均清晰时，即可描绘。

【实验报告】

1. 测量甘草导管的大小。

2. 以显微描绘器绘图法描绘甘草根横切片中一部分的组织，经计算后注明所绘图的放大倍数。

3. 描绘甘草根横切片组织简图。

【思考题】

1. 在显微测量时，为何需要先对目镜量尺进行标化？

2. 徒手绘图法有何缺点？如何克服？

Experiment 3　Microscopical Measurement and Microscopical Drawing

【Objective】

1. To master the methods of microscopical measurement and microscopical drawing.

【Principle】

1. Microscopical measurement scale

Microscopical measurement of fine object is a routine work in microscopical identification of crude drug. Two microscopical measurement scales are required, known as eyepiece micrometer and stage micrometer. Additionally, there is another kind of scale ruled in squares used for counting number and measureing area of object.

The eyepiece micrometeris a fine scale engraved on a disc glass with a diameter of 18～20mm. The scale is 1cm or 0.5cm long and is divided into 50～200 fine divisions. The eyepiece micrometer can be used for measuring length of object directly.

The stage micrometer is a glass slide with a scale engraved at the center. The scale is 1mm long and is divided into 10 and 100 divisions of a millimetre. The stage micrometer can not be used for measuring length of object directly.

2. Microscopical drawing

For microscopical drawing, there are two types of illustration, viz. diagrammatic sketch and detailed drawing.

（1）Diagrammatic sketch：In a diagrammatic sketch, tissues are simply presented with various symbols. General symbols are illustrated below.

（2）Detailed drawing：In a detailed drawing, cells in tissues are depicted in detail, and the characters of each cell including shape, cell wall, pit and striation are reqired to be presented as far as possible. A detailed drawing can be achieved by free－hand drawing or camera lucida－drawing. In addtion, the digital photomicrography device has been developed and popularly applied in the microscopical identification of crude drug, owing to its real－time and high－fidelityadvantages.

【Instruments and Reagents】

Eyepiece micrometer, stage micrometer, drawing eyepiece.

【Materials】

Permanent slide of transverse section of Glycyrrhizae Radix et Rhizoma.

【Experimental Procedures】

1. Determination of eyepiece micrometer

The value of eyepiece micrometer varies with the magnification of optial combinations of eyepiece lens and objective lens. Therefore, the value of one eyepiece division should be determined before microscopical measurement. To do this, put the stage micrometer on the stage and replace the eyepiece lens with eyepiece micrometer. Focus the two micrometer sacles, and make the 0 lines concident. Find out the concidence lines on the right. Then calculate the micron number of 1 eyepiece division, using the following equation.

2. Microscopical measurement

Repalce the stage micrometer with the specimen slide of Glycyrrhizae Radix et Rhizoma, measure the size of an object, i. e. , the diameter of a xylem vessel.

3. Microscopical drawing

Put the specimen slide of Glycyrrhizae Radix et Rhizoma on the stage, observe the whole structure under lower power objective, then observe phloem, cambium and xylemunder high power objective, draw a representative tissue.

（1）Free – hand drawing: Using a pencil, draw the observed image. Drawing while observing, modifying until satisfied.

（2）Camera lucida – drawing: Place the camera lucida into the draw tube, suitably adjust the illumination of both object and paper, so that the pencil appears superimposed on the object, which may thus be traced.

【Assignments】

1. Measure the size of a xylem vessel.

2. Drawin dtaila portion of transverse section of Glycyrrhizae Radix et Rhizoma（under 40 × objective）by the method of camera lucida – drawing, note the magnification after calculation.

3. Sketch the structure of transverse section of Glycyrrhizae Radix et Rhizoma.

【Discussion】

1. Why the value of eyepiece micrometer should be determined before microscopical measurement?

2. What are the drawbacks of free – hand drawing method? How to overcome them?

实验四 生药的显微化学鉴别

【实验目的】

掌握生药显微化学鉴别法的原理和方法。

【实验指导】

生药的显微化学鉴别法兼有显微鉴别和理化鉴别两种方法的内容。其方法是将生药的粉末片或浸出液，置载玻片上，滴加适宜的化学试剂制成临时装片，在显微镜下观察所产生的沉淀、结晶、气泡、溶解、颜色变化等现象，确定细胞壁的组成、细胞后含物的性质、化学成分在生药组织中的分布等，从而达到鉴别生药的目的。

【仪器与试剂】

1. 仪器

显微镜、微量升华装置、水浴锅、切片刀、镊子等。

2. 试剂

间苯三酚试液、浓盐酸、氯化锌碘试液、66% 硫酸、苏丹Ⅲ试液、碘试液、30% 硫酸、稀醋酸、10% α–萘酚乙醇试液、乙醇、稀盐酸、30% 硝酸、碘化铋钾试液、10% 氢氧化钠、1% 三氯化铁试液、5% 氢氧化钡等。

【实验材料】

直立百部（新鲜块根）、生姜（新鲜块根）、山药、蓖麻子、何首乌、穿心莲、沙参（新鲜根）、黄连、黄柏、槟榔、大黄、牡丹皮、斑蝥。

【实验步骤】

1. 细胞壁性质的鉴别

（1）木质化细胞壁 取新鲜直立百部块根作徒手切片，加间苯三酚试液 1～2 滴，稍放置，加浓盐酸 1 滴，加盖玻片，镜检，可见内皮层细胞壁上的凯氏带和凯氏点、导管、纤维等木化的细胞壁因木化程度不同显红色或紫红色。

（2）纤维素细胞壁 取新鲜直立百部块根作徒手切片，加氯化锌碘试液 1～2 滴，稍放置，再加 66% 硫酸 1～2 滴，加盖玻片，镜检，可见纤维素细胞壁显蓝色。

（3）木栓化细胞壁 取新鲜生姜块根作徒手切片，加苏丹Ⅲ试液 1～2 滴，稍放置，加盖玻片，镜检，可见木栓化细胞壁显橘红色、红色或紫红色。

2. 细胞后含物的鉴别

（1）淀粉粒 取山药粉末，用碘试液装片，镜检，淀粉粒显蓝色。

（2）糊粉粒 取蓖麻子胚乳，切成薄片，用碘试液装片，镜检，糊粉粒显棕色或黄棕色。

（3）草酸钙结晶 取何首乌粉末，用 30% 硫酸装片，镜检，可见草酸钙簇晶逐渐溶解，片刻后析出硫酸钙针晶。

（4）碳酸钙结晶　取穿心莲叶作表面制片，用稀醋酸试液装片，镜检，可见钟乳体逐渐溶解，同时产生大量气泡。

（5）菊糖　取沙参根作徒手切片，加 10% α – 萘酚乙醇试液 1～2 滴，66% 硫酸 1 滴，稍加热，镜检，可见菊糖显紫色并很快溶解。

3. 某些化学成分的鉴别

（1）小檗碱　取黄连或黄柏粉末少许，置载玻片上，滴加乙醇 1 滴，放置片刻，使微干，加稀盐酸 1～2 滴，放置 5～10 分钟，加盖玻片，镜检，可见析出的黄色针簇状盐酸小檗碱结晶；若加 30% 硝酸，则可见析出的黄色针簇状硝酸小檗碱结晶。

（2）槟榔碱　取槟榔粉末约 0.5g，置试管中，加水 2ml 及稀盐酸 1 滴，放置片刻，在水浴上加热数分钟，冷却后滤过，取滤液 1 滴，于载玻片上，加碘化铋钾试液 1 滴，即发生浑浊；加盖玻片，镜检，可见石榴红色的球形或方形结晶。

（3）大黄酚、丹皮酚、斑蝥素　有些生药中所含有的某些化学成分，在一定温度下具有升华的性质，如大黄酚、丹皮酚、斑蝥素等。微量升华法即利用这一特性，借助微量升华装置（图 4 – 1），从少量生药中获得升华物，在显微镜下观察其形状、颜色以及化学反应，从而达到鉴别的目的。

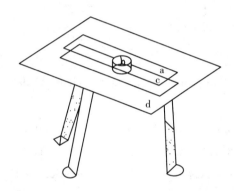

图 4 – 1　微量升华装置

Figure 4 – 1　Microsublimation device

a. 载玻片（glass slide）；b. 金属圈（mental ring）；c. 金属片（mental sheet）；

d. 中有小孔的石棉板（asbesto board with small hole）

取大黄粉末少许于微量升华装置的金属圈内，小火徐徐加热数分钟，可见黄色升华物附着载玻片上；将玻片取下翻转后，镜检，低温升华时可见针状结晶，高温时可见羽毛结晶；滴加 10% 氢氧化钠，结晶溶解而呈红色。

取牡丹皮粉末少许，同上法进行微量升华，镜检，升华物呈长柱形、针状、羽状结晶，滴加 1% 三氯化铁试液，结晶溶解而呈暗紫色。

取斑蝥素粉末少许，同上法进行微量升华，镜检，升华物呈柱形、棱形结晶，滴加 5% 氢氧化钡，可见斑蝥酸钡盐针晶束。

【实验报告】

记录显微化学试验的结果。

【思考题】

生药的显微化学鉴别法有何优点？

Experiment 4　Micro – chemical Identification
of Crude Drugs

【Objective】

To master the method of micro – chemical identification of crude drugs.

【Principle】

Micro – chemical identification involves microscopical identification and chemical test. To do this, place powder or soaking extract of crude drugs on the slide glass, add specific reagents, observe the generated phenomina including precipitation, crystallization, bubbling, dissolution, and color changing, which are of value in identification of composition of the cell wall, cell ergastic substance, distribution of chemical constituents.

【Instruments and Reagents】

1. Instruments

Optical microscope, microsublimation device, water – bath, blade, test tube, tweezers.

2. Reagents

Phloroglucinol TS, concentrated hydrochloric acid, zinc chloride iodine TS, 66% sulphuric acid, Sudan Ⅲ TS, iodine TS, 30% sulphuric acid, dilute acetic acid, 10% α – naphthol ethanol TS, ethanol, dilute hydrochloric acid, 30% nitric acid, potassium iodide TS, 10% sodium hydroxide, 1% ferric chloride TS, 5% barium hydroxide.

【Materials】

Stemonae Radix(fresh root), Zingiberis Rhizoma(fresh rhizome), Dioscoreae Rhizoma, Ricini Semen, Polygoni Multiflori Radix, Andrographitis Herba, Adenophorae Radix, Coptidis Rhizoma, Phellodendri Cortex, Arecae Semen, Rhei Radix et Rhizoma, Moutan Cortex, Mylabris.

【Experimental Procedures】

1. Identification of cell wall

(1)Lignified cell wall: Add 1 ~ 2 drops of phloroglucinol TS to the specimen slide of Stemonae Radix. Allow to stand for a moment, add one drop of concentrated hydrochloric acid, examine under a microscope, the lignified walls of Casparian strip or Casparian dots, vessels, and fibres show a red color or purplish – red color, depending on the extent of lignification.

(2)Cellulose cell wall: Add 1 ~ 2 drops of zine chloride – iodine TS to the specimen slide of Stemonae Radix. Stand for a moment, add 1 ~ 2 drops of 66% sulphuric acid, examine under a microscope, the cellulose walls show a blue or purple color.

(3)Suberized cell wall: Add 1 – 2 drops of Sudan Ⅲ TS to the specimen slide of Zingiberis

Rhizoma. Stand for a moment, examine under a microscope, the suberized cell walls show an orange - red or red color.

2. Identification of cell ergastic substances

(1) Starch granule: Take the powder of Dioscoreae Rhizoma, mount in iodine TS, examine under a microscope, starch granules show a blue or purple color.

(2) Aleurone granules: Take out the endosperm from Ricini Semen, cut into thick slices, mount in iodine TS, examine under a microscope, aleurone granules show a brown or yellowish - brown color.

(3) Crystals of calcium oxalate: Take the powder of Polygoni Multiflori Radix, mount in 30% sulphuric acid, examine under a microscope, crystals of calcium oxalate dissolve gradually, after a moment acicular crystals of calcium sulfate is precipitated.

(4) Crystals of calciumcarbonate: Take the leaf of Andrographitis Herba, prepare a surface specimen slide, mount in dilute acetic acid, examine under a microscope, cystolithsdissolve gradually, meanwhile plenty of bubbles overflow.

(5) Synanthrin: Take Adenophorae Radix, prepare a transverse section of specimen slide, successively add 1 ~ 2 drops of 10% α - naphthol ethanol TS and 66% sulphuric acid, heat slightly, examine under a microscope, synanthrin shows a purpul color and dissolves immidiately.

3. Identification of chemical constituents

(1) Berberine: Take the powder of Coptidis Rhizoma or Phellodendri Cortex on a slide glass, add a drop of ethanol TS, stand for a moment, add 1 ~ 2 drops of dilute hydrochloric acid, stand for 5 ~ 10min, examine under a microscope, the yellow needle clusters of berberine hydrochloride are precipitated; if 30% nitric acid is dropped, the yellow needle clusters of berberine nitrate are precipitated.

(2) Arecoline: Weigh 0.5g of Arecae Semen powder to a test tube, add 2ml of water and a drop of dilute hydrochloric acid, stand for a moment, heat on a waterbath for several minutes, allow to cool and filter, take one drop of filtrate on a a slide glass, add one drop of potassium iodide TS, the solution becomes muddy, examine under a microscope, the square or quadrate yellow garnet crystals are visible.

(3) Chrysophanol, paeonol, and cantharidin: Some chemical constituents in crude drugs, such as chrysophanol, paeonol, and cantharidin, have the property of sublimation. With the aid of microsublimation device, capture the sublimate onto a slide glass, examine under a microscope, the shape, color and chemical reaction of the sublimate are of significance for identification.

Weigh a small amount of Rhei Radix et Rhizoma powder to the metal ring, heat gently for several minutes, yellow sublimates attach to the slide glass. Take down the slide and turn over, examine under a microscope, needle crystalsare visible after low temperature heating, while feathery crystalsare visible after high temperature; add 1 ~ 2 drops of 10% sodium hydroxide, crystals dissolve, show a red color.

Weigh a small amount of Moutan Cortex powder, conduct the procedures as above described, cylindrical, needle and feathery crystals are visible; add 1 ~ 2 drops of 1% ferric chloride TS, crystals dissolve, show a dark purple color.

Weigh a small amount of Mylabris powder, conduct the procedures as above described, pillar and prismatic crystals are visible; add $1 \sim 2$ drops of 5% barium hydroxide, raphides of barium cantharidinate are visible.

【Assignments】

Record the results of micro – chemical tests.

【Discussion】

What are the advanteges of micro – chemical identification?

实验五　生药中各类化学成分的定性鉴别

【实验目的】

1. 掌握生药中糖类、苷类、黄酮类、生物碱、鞣质、氨基酸和蛋白质化学成分的理化性质和定性鉴别反应，并能应用于生药的鉴别。

2. 了解各类化学成分主要鉴别反应的原理。

【实验指导】

生药中含有的化学成分往往具有不同的结构或者基团，可与特定的试剂产生颜色反应或者沉淀反应。可以应用这些反应现象鉴别生药中化学成分的结构。

【仪器与试剂】

1. 仪器

锥形瓶、试管、量筒、烧杯、水浴锅、电炉、超声波清洗机等。

2. 试剂

Fehling 试液（碱性硫酸铜试液）、10%盐酸、10%氢氧化钠、5%α-萘酚试液、浓硫酸、氢氧化钾试液、硫酸亚铁试液、稀盐酸、5%三氯化铁试液、乙醚、1%醋酸镁甲醇溶液、镁粉、浓盐酸、1%三氯化铝甲醇试液、2%红细胞悬浮液、醋酐、三氯化铁-冰醋酸试液、3,5-二硝基苯甲酸乙醇溶液、7%盐酸羟胺甲醇溶液、20%氢氧化钾甲醇溶液、碘化铋钾试液、碘-碘化钾试液、碘化汞钾试液、硅钨酸试液、鞣酸试液、醋酸铅试液、新配制的饱和石灰水溶液、饱和溴水、茚三酮试液、0.5%硫酸铜试液等。

【实验材料】

党参、苦杏仁、槐花、大黄、夹竹桃叶、桔梗、牡丹皮、白芷、柴胡、百部、马钱子、五倍子、儿茶、鹿茸。

【实验步骤】

1. 糖及苷的鉴别

取党参0.5g，剪碎，置50ml锥形瓶中，加蒸馏水10ml，超声处理5分钟，滤过，取滤液分别进行下列试验。

（1）Fehling 反应　取滤液1ml于50ml烧杯中，加 Fehling 试液8ml，置沸水浴加热5分钟，有砖红色沉淀产生，表明含还原糖（注意：反应液应保持蓝色，否则应适当添加 Fehling 试液至蓝色不褪）。上述溶液继续加热5分钟，放冷，滤过，滤液加10%盐酸，使反应液的 pH 为1~2，再在沸水浴加热10分钟（使多糖及苷类等发生水解），放冷，加10%氢氧化钠试液，使反应液呈中性，再加 Fehling 试剂8ml，沸水浴加热数分钟，产生砖红色沉淀，示多糖或苷的存在。

（2）Molish 反应　取滤液1ml于试管中，加5%α-萘酚试液2~3滴，摇匀，倾斜试管，沿管壁缓缓滴加浓硫酸 1ml，轻放试管架上，保持上下两层界面清晰，观察交界处有无紫红色环形成。

2. 氰苷的鉴别

（1）苦味酸钠试纸反应　取苦杏仁粗粉约 0.5g，置具塞试管中，加水适量湿润，管内悬挂一条苦味酸钠试纸，密塞，将试管置 60℃ 水浴中温热，观察试纸逐步由黄色变为砖红色。

（2）普鲁士蓝反应　取苦杏仁粗粉约 0.5g 置试管中，加水少许湿润，立即用滤纸包扎管口，滤纸用 1~2 滴氢氧化钾试液湿润，将试管置 60℃ 水浴温热约 10 分钟后，于试纸上加硫酸亚铁试液 1 滴、稀盐酸和 5% 三氯化铁试液各 1 滴，滤纸即显蓝色。

3. 蒽醌的鉴别

（1）Bornträger's 反应　取大黄粉末 0.1g 于试管中，加 10% 氢氧化钠 2ml，振摇，溶液即呈红色，滤过，滤液加 10% 盐酸使中和，溶液变黄色；加入乙醚 2ml，振摇使之分层，醚液呈黄色，吸取醚液层置另一试管中，加氢氧化钠试液 1ml，振摇后碱液又显红色。

（2）醋酸镁反应　取大黄粉末约 0.2g 于试管中，加乙醇 3ml，超声处理 5 分钟，滤过，滤液加 1% 醋酸镁甲醇溶液 2 滴，振摇后观察，溶液渐呈橙红色。

4. 黄酮的鉴别

取槐米粗粉 0.5g，加乙醇 10ml，超声处理 5 分钟，滤过，得滤液。

（1）盐酸 – 镁粉还原反应　取上述滤液 2ml 于试管中，先滴加浓盐酸 2~3 滴，再加镁粉少许，振摇，产生大量气泡，同时溶液渐变为樱红色。

（2）三氯化铝反应　取上述滤液 2ml 于试管中，加 1% 三氯化铝甲醇溶液 lml，振摇，可见溶液渐变为鲜黄色。

5. 皂苷的鉴别

取桔梗粗粉 1g，置 50ml 锥形瓶中，加生理盐水 15ml，超声处理 5 分钟，滤过，得滤液。

（1）泡沫试验　取上述滤液 2ml，置试管中，密塞或以手指压住管口，强烈振摇数分钟，观察是否产生大量泡沫，放置 10 分钟后，再记录泡沫的高度。

（2）溶血试验　将 2% 红细胞悬浮液滴于载玻片上，盖上盖玻片，置显微镜下，观察红细胞形状，然后于盖玻片边缘滴加桔梗滤液，观察有无溶血现象。如红细胞破裂溶解，为阳性反应。

（3）Libermann 反应　取柴胡粗粉 1g，置锥形瓶中，加 70% 乙醇 10ml，超声处理 5 分钟，滤过，滤液置蒸发皿中，水浴蒸干，放冷，加醋酐 1ml 使溶解，并转入小试管中，沿管壁加浓硫酸 1ml，两液面的交界处显紫红色环。

6. 强心苷的鉴别

取夹竹桃叶粗粉 2g，加 70% 乙醇 15ml，再加 10% 醋酸铅 2ml，超声处理 5 分钟，滤过，得滤液。

（1）Keller – Kiliani 反应（α – 去氧糖反应）　取上述滤液 2ml 于蒸发皿中，水浴蒸干，加三氯化铁 – 冰醋酸试液 1ml 使残渣溶解，并转入小试管中，沿管壁缓缓滴加浓硫酸 lml，观察两液层交界处有棕色环产生，冰醋酸层显蓝绿色。

（2）Kedde's 反应（3,5 – 二硝基苯甲酸反应）　取上述滤液 5ml，加等量新配制的 3,5 – 二硝基苯甲酸乙醇溶液，溶液显紫红色。

7. 香豆素的鉴别

异羟肟酸铁反应取白芷粗粉0.5g，置具塞试管中，加乙醚3ml，超声处理5分钟，静置约20分钟，取上清液1ml于另一试管中，加7%盐酸羟胺甲醇溶液与20%氢氧化钾甲醇溶液各2~3滴，摇匀，置水浴上微热，冷却后，加稀盐酸调节pH至3~4，再加1%三氯化铁乙醇溶液1~2滴，溶液呈紫红色。

8. 生物碱的鉴别

取百部粗粉1g于50ml锥形瓶中，加1%盐酸15ml，超声处理5分钟，滤过；将滤液分装于6支小试管中，每试管1ml，其中一支作为空白对照，其余分别滴加下表5-1中生物碱沉淀剂各2滴，观察沉淀的颜色。

表5-1　生物碱沉淀反应

沉淀试剂	碘化铋钾	碘-碘化钾	碘化汞钾	硅钨酸	鞣酸
沉淀颜色	桔红色	棕色	白色	灰白色	浅棕黄色

9. 鞣质的鉴别

分别取五倍子与儿茶粗粉2g于50ml锥形瓶中，加水20ml，超声处理5分钟，冷却，滤过，五倍子滤液和儿茶滤液分别各置5支试管，依次加入表5-2中试剂，观察溶液颜色及有无沉淀产生。

表5-2　鞣质沉淀/颜色反应

试剂	五倍子（可水解鞣质）	儿茶（缩合鞣质）
醋酸铅试液	乳白色沉淀	淡黄色沉淀，易溶于稀醋酸
新配制的饱和石灰水	青灰色沉淀	棕色或红棕色沉淀
饱和溴水	无沉淀	黄色或橙红色沉淀
三氯化铁试液	溶液显蓝色或蓝黑色并有沉淀	溶液显绿色或绿黑色或沉淀

10. 氨基酸与蛋白质的鉴别

取鹿茸粉末0.1g于试管中，加水约4ml，超声处理5分钟，滤过，得滤液。

（1）茚三酮反应　取滤液1ml于试管中，加新配制的茚三酮试液2滴，水浴加热数分钟，观察颜色反应。另取小滤纸，滴加天花粉溶液1滴，吹干，再滴加茚三酮试剂1滴，用电吹风烘烤，观察颜色变化。

（2）双缩脲反应　取天花粉溶液4ml于试管中，加10%氢氧化钠试液2滴，再加0.5%硫酸铜试液2滴，振摇并静置，观察溶液颜色变化。溶液显蓝色为阳性反应。

【实验报告】

记录各鉴别反应的步骤与结果，并说明反应原理（可用化学反应式表示）。

【思考题】

1. Fehling反应中，水解前后产生砖红色沉淀的主要成分是什么？

2. 怎样鉴别某生药含单糖、多糖或苷类成分？

3. 怎样鉴别生药中是否含有蒽醌类成分？

4. 如何区别某生药所含皂苷是三萜皂苷还是甾体皂苷？

5. 异羟肟酸铁反应开始时，加碱性试剂的作用是什么？

6. 如何确证某一生药中存在生物碱类成分？

7. 如何区别可水解鞣质与缩合鞣质？

8. 如何鉴别生药中存在的是氨基酸还是蛋白质？

Experiment 5　Identification of Main Chemical Constituents in Crude Drugs

【Objective】

1. To master the physio – chemical properties of carbohydrates, glycosides, cyanophoric glycosides, anthraquinones, flavonoids, saponins, cardiac glycosides, alkaloids, tannins, amino acids and proteins in crude drugs.

2. To know the principles of identification reactions.

【Principle】

Chemical constituentsin crude drugs often have different structures or groups that can react with a specific reagent to generate coloringor precipitating phemonia, indicating the presence of chemical constituents.

【Instruments and Reagents】

1. Instruments
Conical flask, beaker, test tube, water bath, ultrasonic cleaner, sodium picrate test paper.

2. Reagents
Fehling TS(basic cuper sulfate), 10% hydrochloric acid, 10% sodium hydroxide, 5% α – naphthol TS, concentratedsulphuric acid, potassium hydroxide TS, ferric sulphate TS, dilute hydrochloric acid, 5% ferric chloride TS, diethyl ether, 1% magnesium acetate TS, magnesium powder, concentrated hydrochloric acid, 1% aluminum chloride methanol TS, 2% erythrocyte suspension, acetic anhydride, ferric chloride glacial acetic acid TS, 3,5 – dinitrobenzoic acid TS, 7% hydroxylamine hydrochloride, bismuth potassium iodide TS, iodine – potassium iodide TS, mercuric potassium iodide TS, silicon tungstic acid TS, tannic acid TS, lead acetate TS, saturated lime aqueous solution(freshely prepared), saturated limit(freshely prepared), ninhydrin TS, 0.5% copper sulfate TS.

【Materials】

Codonopsis Radix, Armeniacae Semen Amarum, Sophorae Flos, Rhei Radix et Rhizoma, Thevetiae Folium, Platycodis Radix, Bupleuri Radix, Angelicae Dahuricae Radix, Stemonae Radix, Galla Chinensis, Catechu, Cervi Pantotrichum Cornu.

【Experimental Procedures】

1. Identification of sugars and glycosides

Cut 0.5g of Codonopsis Radix into fragments to a 50ml conical flask, add 10ml of distilled water, ultrasonicate for 5min, filter.

(1) Fehling test: Add 1ml of filtrate and 8ml Fehling agent in a 50ml beaker, heat on a water bath for 5min, a brick – red precipitate is produced, indicating the presence of reducing sugars. (Note: the reaction system should be maintained blue by adding Fehling agent, if needed). The solution is continued to be heated for 5min, allow to cool, filter, add 10% hydrochloric acid to the filtrate until pH is 1 to 2, heat on a boiling water bath for 10min, allow to cool, add 10% sodium hydroxide to neutralize the reaction solution, then add 8ml of Fehling TS, heat on a boiling water bath for several minutes, a brick – red precipitate is produced, indicating the presence of glycosides.

(2) Molish test: Add 1ml of filtrate and 2 ~ 3 drops of α – naphthol TS to a test tube, shake well, slowly add 1ml of concentrated sulfuric acid along the tubal wall, keep the interface clear, observe whether a violet – red ring is produced at the junction.

2. Identification of cyanogenic glycosides

(1) Sodium picrate test: Weigh 0.5g of Armeniacae Semen Amarumcoarse powder to a test tube stopped with a cork, moisten with several drops of water, hang a strip of sodium picrate test paper, stopper tightly, heat the tube on a 60℃ water bath. Test paper changes from yellow to brick – red gradually.

(2) Prussian blue test: Weigh 0.5g of Armeniacae Semen Amarumcoarse powder to a tube stopped with a cork, moisten with several drops of water, then wrap the mouth of the tube with filter paper, moisten the filter paper with 1 ~ 2 drops of potassium hydroxide, heat the tube on a 60℃ water bath for 10min, add a drop of ferrous sulfate, 5% chloride ferric and dilute hydrochloric acid successively. Filter paper shows blue color.

3. Identification of anthraquinones

(1) Bornträger's test: Weigh 0.1g of Rhei Radix et Rhizoma powder to a test tube, add 2ml of 10% potassium hydroxide, shake well. The solution becomes red. Filter, neutralize with 10% hydrochloric acid, the solution becomes yellow. Add 2ml of diethyl ether, shake, the ether layer becomes yellow. Transfer the ether solution into another test tube, add 1ml of potassium hydroxide, shake, the alkaline solution turn red again.

(2) Magnesium acetate test: Weigh 0.2g of Rhei Radix et Rhizoma coarse powder to a test tube, add 3ml of ethanol, ultrasonicate for 5min, filter, add 2 drops of 1% magnesium acetate TS to the filtrate, shake, the solution becomes orange – red.

4. Identification of flavonoids

Weigh 0.5g of Sophorae Flos coarse powder to a 50ml conical flask, add 10ml of ethanol, ultrasonicate for 5min, filter.

(1) HCl – Mg reduction reaction: Take 2ml of filtrate into a test tube, add 2 – 3 drops of concentrated hydrochloric acidand a small amount of magnesium powder, a large number of bubbles appear after shaking, and the solution becomes cherry red.

（2）AlCl₃ reaction：Take 2ml of filtrate into a test tube，add 1ml of 1% aluminum chloride methanol TS，the solution becomes bright yellow after shaking.

5. Identification of saponins

Weigh 1g of Platycodis Radix coarse powder to a 50ml of conical flask，add 15ml of normal saline，ultrasonicate for 5min，filter.

（1）Foam test：Take 2ml of filtrate to a test tube，stopper tightly. Shake violently for several minutes，lots of foams appear. Stand for 10min，then compare the height of foams before and after standing.

（2）Hematolysis test：Drop 2% erythrocyte suspension on a slide glass，observe the shape of erythrocyte under microscope. Then drop Platycodis Radix filtrate to the edge of slide glass，observe whether hematolysis response generates. The dissolution of erythrocyte proves a positive reaction.

（3）Libermann test：Weigh 1g of Platycodis Radix coarse powder to a conical flask，add 10ml of 70% ethanol，ultrasonicate for 5min，filter. Evaporate the filtrate to dryness，allow to cool，dissolve the residue in 1ml of acetic anhydride and transfer to a small tube，add 1ml of concentrated sulfuric acid along tube wall，a violet－red loop appear at the junction of two layers.

6. Identification of cardiac glycosides

To 2g of Thevetiae Folium coarse powder，add 15ml of 70% ethanol and 2ml of 10% lead acetate solution，ultrasonicate for 5min，filter.

（1）Keller－Kiliani test：Evaporate 2ml of filtrate to dryness，dissolve the residue in 1ml of 5% ferric chloride TS，and transfer to a small tube，add 1ml of concentrated sulfuric acid along tube wall，a brown loop appear at the junction of two layers，the glacial acetic acid layershows blue－green color.

（2）Kedde's test：To 5ml of filtrate，add 5ml of fresheley prepared 3,5－dinitro－benzoic acid in ethanol，the solution becomes voilet－red.

7. Identification of coumarins

Ferric hydroxamic test：Weigh 0.5g of Angelicae Dahuricae Radix coarse powderto a stopperedtube，add 3ml of ether，ultrasonicate for 5min，stand for 20min. Take 1ml of supernatant to another tube，add 2 or 3 drops of 7% hydroxylamine hydrochloride in methanol and 20% potassium hydroxidein methanol succesively，shake，heat on a water bath，allow to cool，add hydrochloric acid to adjust pH to 3 or 4，then add 1 or 2 drops of 1% ferric chlorideTS，the solution becomes voilet－red.

8. Identification of alkaloids

Weigh 1g of Stemonae Radix coarse powder to a conical flask，add 15ml of 1% hydrochloric acid，ultrasonicate for 5min，filter，transfer the filtrate into six test tubes respectively，1ml per tube. Using one tube as blank control，2 drops of alkaloid－precipitantreagents are added to the other five tubes as Table 5－1. Observe the color of precipitate.

Table 5－1 Precipitation reaction of alkaloids

Precipitantreagent	Bismuth potassium iodide TS	Iodine－potassium iodide TS	Mercuric potassium iodide TS	Silicon tungstic acid TS	Ttannic acid TS
Color	Orange－red	Brown	White	Greywish－white	Light brown－yellow

9. Identification of tannins

Weigh 2g of Galla Chinensis or Catechu coarse powder two a conical flask, add 20ml of water. Ultrasonicate for 5min and filter. Transfer the filtrates of Galla Chinensis or Catechu to five test tubes, add the reagents successively as Table 5 – 2. Observe the color change and precipitate.

Table 5 – 2　Color change and precipitation reaction of tannins

Reagent	Galla Chinensis (Hydrolysable tannins)	Catechu (Condensed tannins)
Lead acetateTS	Cream white precipitate; undissolvable in dilute acetic acid	Light yellow precipitate; dissolvabe in dilute acetic acid
Saturated lime aqueous solution	Green – gray precipitate	Brown or reddish – brown precipitate
Saturated limit	No precipitate	Yellow or orange – red precipitate
Ferric chloride TS	Blue or blue – black solution; having precipitate	Green or green – black solution; havingprecipitate

10. Identification of amino acids and proteins

Weigh 0. 1g of Cervi Pantotrichum Cornu powder to a test tube, add 4ml of water. Ultrasonicate for 5min and filter.

（1）Ninhydrinreaction：Take 1ml of filtrate into a test tube, add 2 drops of freshly preparedninhydrin TS, heat on a water bath for several minutes, observe the color change. Add 1 drop of the filtrate to a piece of small filter paper, blow to dryness, then add 1 drop of ninhydrin TS, blow to dryness with a hair drier, observe the color change. The blue solution provesa positive reaction.

（2）Biuretreaction：Take 4ml of filtrate into a test tube, add 2 drops of 10% potassium hydroxide TS and 0. 5% copper sulfate TS successively, shake and stand. Observe the color change. The blue solution provesa positive reaction.

【Assignments】

1. Record the procedures and results of identification tests, and explain the principles of chemical reactions by using the chemical formulas.

【Discussion】

1. In Fehling test, what're the main constituents for resulting in cuprous oxide precipitation before and after the hydrolysis?

2. How to identify the monosaccharides, polysaccharides and glycosides in some crude drugs?

3. How to identify the anthraquinone constituents in crude drugs?

4. How to distinguish thetriterpenoid saponins and steroidal saponins?

5. At the beginning of the reaction of ferric hydroxamic test, what's the purpose of adding alkalinity agent?

6. How to confirm the presence of alkaloids in crude drugs?

7. How to distinguish hydrolysable tannins and condensed tannins?

8. How to identify the presence of amino acids or proteins in crude drugs?

实验六 生药薄层色谱鉴别

【实验目的】

掌握生药的薄层色谱鉴别方法。

【实验指导】

薄层色谱法又称薄层层析法（thinlayercharomatography，TLC），系将供试品溶液点于薄层板上，在展开容器内用展开剂展开，使供试品所含目标成分分离。TLC 中常用比移值（R_f）来表示各斑点/条带在色谱中的移行位置。

$$R_f = \frac{基线至展开斑点中心的距离}{基线至展开剂前沿的距离}$$

在相同的展开条件下，同一化合物在薄层板上的 R_f 相同，可用于生药的定性鉴别。

其操作方法一般包括以下 5 个步骤：

1. 供试品溶液的制备

中药成分复杂，目标成分的分离和检测往往容易受到干扰，在选择合适的溶剂进行目标成分提取的同时，需要适度的富集或净化，如液 – 液萃取、固 – 液萃取法等。

2. 点样

通常在洁净干燥的环境，用专用毛细管或配合半自动或自动点样器将样品点样于薄层板上，点样体积一般为 0.5 ~ 10μl，可采用点状点样或条带状点样。常见的薄层板有硅胶板、聚酰胺板、氧化铝板等，有市售薄层板（普通或高效板）和自制薄层板。点样时注意勿损伤薄层板表面。

3. 展开

将点样后的薄层板放入展开缸中，确保样品斑点在展开剂液面 5mm 以上。展开前如需要溶剂蒸气预平衡，可在展开缸中加入适量的展开剂，密闭，一般保持 15 ~ 30 分钟，或在展开缸的内侧放置与展开缸内径同样大小的滤纸使展开缸达到溶剂蒸气饱和的状态。除另有规定外，一般上行展开 8 ~ 15cm，高效薄层板上行展开 5 ~ 8cm。溶剂前沿达到规定的展距，取出薄层板，晾干，待检测。必要时，可进行二次展开或双向展开。

4. 显色与检视

供试品中含有在可见光下显色的成分时可直接在日光下检视，也可用喷雾法或浸渍法以适宜的显色剂显色或加热显色后在日光下检视。有荧光或遇某些试剂可激发荧光的物质可在 365nm 紫外光下观察荧光色谱。对于在可见光下无色，但在紫外光下有吸收的成分可用带有荧光剂的硅胶板（如硅胶 GF254 板），在 254nm 紫外光下观察荧光板面上的荧光猝灭物质形成的色谱。

5. 色谱记录与识别

薄层色谱图像一般可采用摄像设备拍摄，以光学照片或电子图像的形式保存。也可用薄层扫描仪扫描记录相应的色谱图。对所得色谱的识别，主要是观察供试品溶液所显主斑点的颜色（或荧光）和位置是否与对照品溶液的斑点一致。

【仪器与试剂】

1. 仪器

超声波清洗机、高效硅胶 G 薄层板、双槽展开缸、电子天平、紫外分析仪、具塞锥形瓶等。

2. 试剂

环己烷、乙酸乙酯、异丙醇、甲醇、三乙胺、浓氨试液、蒸馏水、盐酸黄连碱对照品、盐酸表小檗碱对照品、盐酸小檗碱对照品、盐酸巴马汀对照品等。

【实验材料】

黄连（包括味连、雅连和云连）及黄连对照药材。

【实验步骤】

1. 溶液的制备

（1）供试品溶液　取黄连药材粉末 0.25g，加甲醇 25ml，密塞，超声处理 30 分钟，滤过，取上清液作为供试品溶液。

（2）对照药材溶液　另取黄连对照药材 0.25g，同法制成对照药材溶液。

（3）对照品溶液　分别取盐酸黄连碱对照品、盐酸表小檗碱对照品、盐酸小檗碱对照品和盐酸巴马汀对照品，加甲醇制成每 1ml 各含 0.5mg 的溶液，作为对照品溶液。

2. 点样、展开

吸取上述溶液各 2μl，分别点于同一高效硅胶 G 薄层板上，以环己烷 – 乙酸乙酯 – 异丙醇 – 甲醇 – 水 – 三乙胺（3：3.5：1：1.5：0.5：1）为展开剂；展开前，于展开缸一侧放展开剂，另一侧放等体积氨水，预平衡 20 分钟。展开，取出，晾干。

3. 检视

置紫外光灯（365nm）下检视。供试品色谱中，在与对照药材和对照品色谱相应位置上，显相同颜色的斑点（图 6 – 1）。

【实验报告】

记录黄连薄层色谱鉴别的操作步骤，绘出薄层色谱图，并计算黄连碱、表小檗碱、小檗碱、巴马汀的 R_f 值。

【思考题】

1. 在薄层色谱中，影响 R_f 值的因素有哪些？

2. 在生药薄层色谱鉴别中，采用对照药材作为对照，有何优势？

Experiment 6   Thin Layer Chromatographic Identification of Crude Drugs

【Objective】

To master the method of thin layer chromatographic identification of crude drugs.

【Principle】

Thin layer chromatography is a method that the test solution is applied onto a thin layer plate, and developed with developing solvent in a chamber, so as to chromatograph the target constituent. R_f value is often used in TLC to indicate the transition position of each spot in the chromatography.

$$R_f = \frac{\text{Distance from the base line to the center of the target spot}}{\text{Distance from the base line to the leading edge of the developing solvent}}$$

Under the same TLC condition, the compound has the same R_f, which can be used for qualitative identification of crude drugs.

A typical TLC includes the following five steps:

1. Preparation of test solution

A crude drug is often chemically complicated, isolationand detection of target constituent is easily interfered by other co – existing constituents. In this context, appropriate enrichment or purification steps are needed, such as liquid – liquid extraction, solid – liquid extraction method, etc.

2. Application of test solution

Usually in a clean and dry environment, the test solution is applied onto the thin laminate with special capillary and semi – automatic or automatic sampler, as a small spot or a narrow band. The loading volume is $0.5 \sim 10\mu l$. The glass plate is usually coated with silica Gel or alumin a, or the sheet is coated with polyamide. On applying, do not damage the surface of coated plate.

3. Development

Place the plate in a chromatographic chamber, and ensure that the spots are at least 5mm above the surface of the development solvent. If needed, the chamber can be pre – saturated with the development solvent for $15 \sim 30$min, or can be pre – saturated with the filter paper wet with the development solvent. Unless otherwise stated, upwardly develope over a path of $8 \sim 15$cm, or $5 \sim$ 8cm for a HPTLC. Once the front of development solvent reaches the distance, remove the plate from the chamber and dry in air. If necessary, develop two times or in two dimensions.

4. Visualization and examination

The constituents that show color under visible light can be examined directly in the sunlight, other constituents can be examined by spray method or immersion method with a suitable chromogenic agent. The constituents that have fluorescence property or excite fluorescence by certain reagents can be examined under ultraviolet light at 365nm. For the constituents that are colorless under visible light but have absorption under ultraviolet light, silica gel plate with fluorescence agent (such as silica gel GF254 plate) can be used to examine the chromatography formed by fluorescence quenching substances on the surface of the fluorescence plate under ultraviolet light at 254nm.

5. Chromatogram recording and recognition

Thin layer chromatography images can generally be taken by camera equipment, stored in the form of optical photos or electronic images, or can be scanned by thin layer scanner to record the corresponding chromatogram. The chromatograms obtained with the test and reference solutions are compared in terms of color and position of the main spots.

【Instruments and Reagents】

1. Instruments

Ultrasonic cleaner, silica gel G pre – coated plate, a twin trough chamber, electronic balance, ultraviolet spectrograph, stoppered flask.

2. Reagents

Cyclohexane, ehylacetae, isopropanol, methanol, water, triethylamine, strong ammonia TS, coptisine hydrochloride CRS, epiberberine hydrochloride CRS, berberine hydrochloride CRS, and palmatine hydrochloride CRS.

【Materials】

Coptidis Rhizome, Coptidis Rhizome reference crude drug.

【Experimental Procedures】

1. Preparation of solutions

(1) Test solution: Weigh 0.25g of the Coptidis Rhizome powder, add 25ml of methanol, ultrasonicate for 30min, filter and use the filtrate as the test solution.

(2) Reference crude drug solution: Prepare a solutuion of 0.25g of Coptidis Rhizome reference crude drug in the same manner as the reference crude drug solution.

(3) Reference solution: Dissolve coptisine hydrochloride CRS, epiberberine hydrochloride CRS, berberine hydrochloride CRS, and palmatine hydrochloride CRS in methanol to produce a solution containing 0.5mg per ml as the reference solution, respectively.

2. Application and development

Carry out the method for TLC, using silica gel G as the coating substance and a mixture of cyclohexane, ehylacetae, isopropanol, methanol, water, and triethylamine (3:3.5:1:1.5:0.5:1) as the mobile phase. Apply separately to the plate 2μl of each of the above solutions. After developing in a chamber pre – equilibrating with vapour of strong ammonia TS for 20min, and removal of the plate, dry in air.

3. Examination

Examine under ultraviolet light at 365nm. The fluorescent spots in the chromatogarm obtained with the test solution correspond in position and color to the fluorescent spots in the chromatogram obtained with the reference crude drug solution and the reference solutuons.

【Assignments】

Desribe the experimental procedure of TLC, depict the TLC chromatogram, and calculate the R_f values of coptisine, epiberberine, berberine and palmatine.

【Discussion】

1. What are the main factors that affect R_f value of a constituent?

2. What are the advantages of employing a reference crude drug in TLC identification?

实验七　生药水分及灰分测定

【实验目的】

1. 掌握生药水分、灰分测定方法。
2. 了解生药中水分、总灰分与酸不溶性灰分测定的意义。

【实验指导】

生药中水分含量与其质量密切相关。水分含量过高，易发生霉变、虫蛀等变质现象。生药中水分测定常用烘干法、甲苯法、减压干燥法等。

为了保证生药不含过多的泥土、砂石等无机杂质，需要测定其灰分，包括总灰分与酸不溶性灰分。当生药的总灰分超过生理灰分（将生药加热灰化后，细胞壁和细胞内的无机物质形成的灰烬）的正常限度时，说明有其他无机杂质掺杂。对于生理灰分含量较高的生药，特别是含草酸钙较多的生药，可测定酸不溶性灰分，以便更准确反映该生药中泥砂等无机物质的混杂程度。因此，灰分的测定对于保证生药纯度具有重要意义。

【仪器与试剂】

1. 仪器
称量瓶、烘箱、电子天平、干燥器、分液漏斗、水分测定器、坩埚、马弗炉、无灰滤纸等。

2. 试剂
甲苯、稀盐酸等。

【实验材料】

大青叶、当归、大黄。

【实验步骤】

1. 烘干法测定水分
取大青叶碎片（直径不超过 3mm）约 5g，平铺于干燥至恒重的扁形称量瓶中，厚度不超过 5mm，精密称定重量（W_1），打开瓶盖在 100～105℃ 干燥 5 小时，将瓶盖盖好，移置干燥器中，冷却 30 分钟，精密称定重量，再在上述温度干燥 1 小时，冷却，称重，至连续两次称重的差异不超过 5mg 为止（W_2）。根据减失的重量，按照式（7-1）计算样品中含有水分的百分数。

$$生药中水分含量(\%) = \frac{W_1 - W_2}{W_1} \times 100\% \qquad (7-1)$$

2. 甲苯法测定水分
（1）洗净全部仪器，置干燥箱内烘干，备用。
（2）将甲苯置分液漏斗中，加少量水充分振摇，放置，分去水层，甲苯蒸馏后备用。

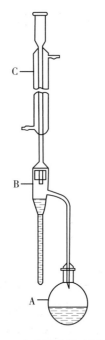

图 7 – 1　水分测定器（甲苯法）

Figure 7 – 1　Water – determining instrument（toluene method）

A. 圆底烧瓶（round – bottomed flask）；

B. 水分测定管（moisture measuring tube）；

C. 直形冷凝管（straight condenser tube）

（3）取当归粗粉适量（相当于含水量 2～4ml），精密称定，置 A 瓶中，加甲苯约 200ml，必要时加玻璃珠数粒，将水分测定器按图 7 – 1 连接，自冷凝管顶端加入甲苯，至充满 B 管的狭细部分。将 A 瓶置电热套中或用其他适宜方法缓缓加热，待甲苯开始沸腾时，调节温度，使每秒钟馏出 2 滴。待水分完全馏出，即测定管刻度部分的水量不再增加时，将冷凝管内部先用适量甲苯冲洗，再用饱蘸甲苯的长刷或其他适宜的方法，将管壁上附着的甲苯推下，继续蒸馏 5 分钟，放冷至室温，拆卸装置，如有水黏附在 B 管上，可用蘸甲苯的铜丝推下，放置，使水分与甲苯完全分离。读取水量，并按照式（7 – 2）换算成样品中含有水分的百分数（V/W）。

$$生药中水分含量（\%）=\frac{水量（ml）}{样品重量（g）}\times100\%$$

$$(7-2)$$

3. 总灰分的测定

取大黄粗粉 3～5g，置已炽灼至恒重的坩埚中，精密称定重量，缓缓炽灼，注意避免燃烧，至完全炭化时，逐渐升高温度至 500～600℃，使完全灰化并至恒重。根据残渣重量，按照式（7 – 3）计算大黄中含灰分的百分数。

$$生药中总灰分含量（\%）=\frac{残渣重}{供试品重量}\times100\%$$

$$(7-3)$$

4. 酸不溶性灰分的测定

取上项所得的灰分，在坩埚中小心加入稀盐酸约 10ml，用表面皿覆盖坩埚，置水浴上加热 10 分钟，表面皿用热水 5ml 冲洗，洗液并入坩埚中，用无灰滤纸滤过，坩埚内的残渣用水洗于滤纸上，并洗涤至洗液不显氯化物反应为止。滤渣连同滤纸移至同一坩埚中，干燥，炽灼至恒重。根据残渣重量，按照式（7 – 4）计算供试品中含酸不溶性灰分的百分数。

$$生药中酸不溶性灰分含量（\%）=\frac{酸处理并烧灼后残渣重量}{供试品重量}\times100\%\qquad(7-4)$$

【实验报告】

1. 分别记录大青叶与当归的水分测定实验步骤，并计算水分含量。
2. 记录灰分测定实验步骤，计算大黄中总灰分与酸不溶性灰分的含量。

【思考题】

1. 干燥失重与水分的含义有何不同？
2. 总灰分和生理灰分的含义有何不同？

Experiment 7　Determination of Water and Ash in Crude Drugs

【Objective】

1. To master the determination methods of water and ash in crude drugs.
2. To know the significance of determination of water and ash in crude drugs.

【Principle】

The water content in crude drug is closely related with its quality. Those crude drugs containing excessive water are prone to go musty or get wormy. The determination methods of water content in crude drug conclude drying method, toluene method and vacuum drying method, etc.

To ensure the crude drug does not contain excessive inorganic foreign matters, such as soil and sandstone, it is necessary to determine the contents of total ash and acid – insoluble ash. When the content of total ash far exceeds the normal limit of physiological ash(origing from the inorganic substances existing in cell walls and cells after heating and ashing the crude drug), it is indicated that the crude drug is adulterated with inorganic foreign substances. For those crude drugs containing high content of physiological ash, especially those containing plenty of calcium oxalate, acid – insoluble ash should be determined so as to accurately reflect the adulteration degree. Consequently, ash determination is significance for ensuring the purity of crude drug.

【Instruments and Reagents】

1. Instruments

Volumetric flask, oven, electronic balance, desicator, separating funnel, water – determining instrument, crucible, Muffle furnace, ashless filter paper.

2. Reagents

Toluene, dilute hydrochloric acid.

【Materials】

Isatidis Folium, Angelicae Sinensis Radix, Rhei Radix et Rhizoma.

【Experimental Procedures】

1. Determination of the water content by drying method

Weigh 5g of Isatidis Folium piece(less than 3mm in diameter)to a flat volumetric flask, spread out to form a smooth layer not exceeding 10mm in thickness, and accurately weigh(W_1). Dry in an oven at $100 \sim 105\,^{\circ}\!C$ for 5h after removal of the stopper. Stopper the flask promptly and allow to cool in a desiccator for 30min. Weigh accurately and dry again for 1h, cool and weigh. Repeat the operation until the difference between two successive weightings is not more than 5mg(W_2).

37

Calculate the percentage content of water according to the following formula.

$$\text{Content of water}(\%) = \frac{W_1 - W_2}{W_1} \times 100\% \qquad (7-1)$$

2. Determination of the water content by toluene method

（1）Wash all the instruments, dry in an oven.

（2）Place the toluene in a separating funnel, add a small amount of water and shake well, stand and separate the water layer, and distill the toluene for use.

（3）Weigh accurately a quantity of the Angelicae Sinensis Radix power（equivalent to the quantity of crude drug containing about 2 ~ 4ml of water）to the flask A. Add about 200ml of toluene and a few glass beads if necessary. Assemble the water – determing instrument as Figure 7 – 1 and fill the receiving tube B with toluene through the top of condenser until the graduated portion is full. Heat the flask A gently. When toluene begins to boil, adjust the temperature to generate the distillate at a rate of 2 drops per second. When the volume of water in the receiving tube does not increase any more, rinse the inside of condenser with toluene and push down the toluene adhering to the wall with a brush or other suitable tools. Continue distillation for 5min. Cool to room temperature and disconnect the instruments. Push down any droplet of water adhering to the wall of the receiving tube with a copper wire wetted with toluene. Stand until water is completely separated from toluene in the receiving tube. Record the volume of distilled water and calculate the percentage of water according to the following formula.

$$\text{Content of water}(\%) = \frac{\text{the volume of water}(ml)}{\text{the weight of sample}(g)} \times 100\% \qquad (7-2)$$

3. Determination of the total ash

Weigh accurately 3 ~ 5g of Rhei Radix et Rhizoma power to a tared crucible, ignite slowly untill the sample is completely carbonized. Keep from burning with care. The temperature is increased gradually to 500 ~ 600℃. Incinerate to constant weight and the ash is carbon – free. Calculate the percentage of ash according to the following formula.

$$\text{Content of total ash}(\%) = \frac{\text{the volume of air – died drug}(ml)}{\text{the weight of sample}(g)} \times 100\% \qquad (7-3)$$

4. Determination of the acid – insoluble ash

Place the above obtained ash in a crucible, add 10ml of dilute hydrochloric acid, covered with a watch glass. Heat on a water bath for 10min. Rinse the watch glass with 5ml of hot water and combine the rinsing solution to crucible. Filter with an ashless filter paper, transfer the residue to the filter paper with water, wash untill the filtrate produces negative reaction to chloride. Transfer the filter paper together with the residue to the crucible, dry and ignite to constant weight. Calculate the percentage of acid – insoluble ash according to the following formula.

$$\text{Content of acid – insoluble ash}(\%) = \frac{\text{the weight of residue dealt}}{\text{the weight of sample}(g)} \times 100\% \qquad (7-4)$$

【Assignments】

1. Record the procedures of water determination for Isatidis Folium and Angelicae Sinensis Radix respectively, and calculate the water contents.

2. Record the procedures of ash determination for Rhei Radix et Rhizoma, calculate the contents of total ash and acid – insoluble ash.

【Discussion】

1. What is the difference between loss on drying and water content?
2. What is the difference between total ash and physiological ash?

实验八　生药挥发油及浸出物测定

【实验目的】

1. 掌握生药挥发油及浸出物测定的方法。
2. 了解生药中挥发油、浸出物含量测定的意义。

【实验指导】

挥发油是一类具有芳香气味的油状液体的总称，可随水蒸气蒸馏，在常温下易挥发，其相对密度一般在 0.850～1.065 之间，除少数挥发油相对密度大于 1.0 外（如丁香油、桂皮油等），大部分生药所含挥发油相对密度小于 1.0。根据挥发油的相对密度大小不同，挥发油的测定有甲、乙两种方法。甲法适用于测定相对密度在 1.0 以下的挥发油，乙法适用于相对密度在 1.0 以上的挥发油。

对于有效成分尚不明确或尚无精确定量方法的生药，一般可根据已知成分的溶解性能，选用适宜的溶剂，提取并测定生药中可溶性浸出物的含量，用以表示该生药的质量。包括水溶性浸出物测定法、醇溶性浸出物测定法和挥发性醚浸出物测定法。供测定的生药样品粉末除另有规定外，应能通过二号筛，并混合均匀。

【仪器与试剂】

1. 仪器

烧瓶、挥发油测定器、回流冷凝管、电热套、电子天平、锥形瓶、蒸发皿、水浴锅、烘箱、干燥器、索氏提取器、容量瓶等。

2. 试剂

二甲苯、乙醇、乙醚、蒸馏水等。

【实验材料】

薄荷、巴戟天、续断、连翘、杜仲、独活。

【实验步骤】

1. 挥发油的测定

甲法：取薄荷（约 5mm 的碎段）适量（约相当于含挥发油 0.5～1.0ml），称定重量，置烧瓶中，每 100g 供试品加水 600ml 与玻璃珠数粒，振摇混合后，连接挥发油测定器与回流冷凝管（图 8-1）。自冷凝管上端加水使充满挥发油测定器的刻度部分，并溢流入烧瓶时为止，置电热套中或其他适宜的方法缓缓加热至沸，并保持微沸约 3 小时，至测定器中油量不再增加，停止加热；放置片刻，开启测定器下端的活塞，将水缓缓放出，至油层上端到达刻度 0 线上方约 5mm 处为止。放置 1 小时以上，再开启活塞使油层下降至上端恰与刻度 0 线平齐，读取挥发油体积，并按照式 8-1 计算样品中含挥发油的百分数（V/W）。

$$样品中挥发油的含量（\%）=\frac{测得的挥发油体积（ml）}{样品重量（g）}\times100\% \qquad (8-1)$$

乙法：取水约300ml与玻璃珠数粒，置烧瓶中，连接挥发油测定器（图8-1）。自测定器上端加水充满刻度部分，并溢流入烧瓶时为止，再用移液管加入二甲苯1ml，然后连接回流冷凝管。将烧瓶内容物加热至沸腾，并继续蒸馏，其速度以保持冷凝管的中部呈冷却状态为度。30分钟后停止加热，放置15分钟以上，读取二甲苯的体积。然后照甲法取供试品适量，依法测定，自油层体积中减去二甲苯的体积，即为挥发油体积，再计算供试品中含挥发油的百分数，计算公式见式（8-2）。

样品中挥发油的含量（%）

$$=\frac{油层体积（ml）-二甲苯体积（ml）}{样品重量（g）}\times100\% \qquad (8-2)$$

2. 浸出物的测定

（1）水溶性浸出物的测定

①冷浸法：取巴戟天粗粉约4g，称定重量，置250ml锥形瓶中，精密加入蒸馏水100ml，密塞冷浸，前6小时内时时振摇，再静置18小时；用干燥滤器迅速滤过，精密吸取滤液20ml，置于已干燥至恒重的蒸发皿中，在水浴上蒸干，于105℃干燥3小时，移置干燥器中，冷却30分钟，迅速精密称定重量，按干燥品计算生药中含水溶性浸出物的百分数。

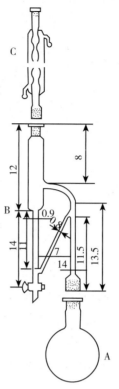

图8-1 挥发油测定装置（长度单位为cm）

Figure 8-1 Apparatus for the determination of volatile oil（lengthunit：cm）

A. 圆底烧瓶（round-bottomed flask）；

B. 挥发油测定器（recogizer of volatile oils）；

C. 球形冷凝管（spherical condenser）

②热浸法：同上法取续断粉末4g于250ml锥形瓶中，精密加入蒸馏水100ml，塞紧，称定重量，静置1小时后，连接冷凝管，加热至沸腾，并保持微沸1小时，放冷后，取下锥形瓶，密塞，称定重量，用水补足减失的重量，摇匀，用干燥滤器滤过。精密吸取滤液25ml，置已干燥至恒重的蒸发皿中，在水浴上蒸干，于105℃干燥3小时，移置干燥器中，冷却30分钟，迅速精密称重，按干燥品计算生药中含水溶性浸出物的百分数。

（2）醇溶性浸出物的测定

醇溶性浸出物的测定亦有冷浸法和热浸法两种，其测定方法与水溶性浸出物的测定法相同，只是用不同浓度的乙醇或甲醇代替水为溶媒。

①冷浸法：取连翘粉末约4g，称定重量，照水溶性浸出物的冷浸法测定，以65%乙醇代替水。

②热浸法：取杜仲粉末约4g，称定重量，照水溶性浸出物的热浸法测定，以75%乙醇代替水。

$$水（醇）溶性浸出物（\%）=\frac{（浸出物及蒸发皿重-蒸发皿重）\times加水（醇）体积}{供试品的重量\times量取滤液的体积}\times100\%$$

$$(8-3)$$

（3）醚溶性浸出物的测定

取独活粉末约2g（通过四号筛），在五氧化二磷干燥器中放置48小时，称定重量，置100ml索氏提取器中，加乙醚70ml，水浴加热回流提取4小时，放冷，过滤，以少量乙醚冲洗烧瓶及回流器，洗液与滤液合并至100ml容量瓶中，加乙醚至刻度，摇匀。精密量取50ml置已干燥至恒重的蒸发皿中，水浴低温蒸去乙醚，移至五氧化二磷干燥器中放置24小时，取出，迅速精密称重，计算样品中含醚溶性浸出物的含量。

$$挥发性醚浸出物（\%）= \frac{干燥前浸出物及蒸发皿重 - 干燥后浸出物及蒸发皿重}{供试品的重量} \times 100\%$$

$$(8-4)$$

【实验报告】

记录生药挥发油和浸出物的测定步骤，并计算含量。

【思考题】

测定挥发油的过程中，影响测定结果的因素有哪些？

Experiment 8　Determination of Volatile Oils and Extractives

【Objective】

1. To master the methods for determination of volatile oils and extractives in crude drugs.

2. To know the significance for determination of volatile oils and extractives in crude drugs.

【Principle】

Volatile oil is a generic term for a kind of aromatic oily liquid, which can be distilled with steam and is volatile at room temperature. Its relative density is generally between 0.850 and 1.065. Except for a few volatile oils whose relative density is heavier than 1.0 (e.g. clove oil and cinnamon oil, etc.), the relative density of volatile oils contained in most crude drug is lighter than 1.0. According to the relative density of volatile oils, there are two determination methods. Method A is applicable to volatile oils with relative density lighter than 1.0, and Method B is applicable to volatile oils with relative density heavier than 1.0.

For those crude drugs whose effective constituents remain unknown or cannot be measured precisely, their quality can be evaluated by determination of the soluble extractives, including water - soluble extractives, alcohol - soluble extractives and ether - soluble extractives.

Unless other stated, the materials should be pulverized to pass through a No. 2 sieve, and well - mixed.

【Instruments and Reagents】

1. Instruments

Flask, apparatus for dermination of volatile oils, reflux condenser, electric heating jacket, electronic balance, conical flask, evaporating dish, water bath, oven, desiccator, Soxhlet extractor, volumetric flask.

2. Reagents

Xylene, ethanol, ethyl ether, distilled water.

【Materials】

Menthae Herba, Morindae Officinalis Radix, Dipsaci Radix, Forsythiae Fructus, Eucommiae Cortex, Angelicae Pubescentis Radix.

【Experimental Procedures】

1. Determination of volatile oils

Method A：Weigh accurately proper quantity of Menthae Herb fragments (5mm in diameter) (equivalent to the weight of crude drug containing 0. 5 ~ 1. 0ml of volatile oils) to flask A. Add 600ml of water per 100 g of the drug and a few glass beads, shake and mix well. Assembly the three parts of apparatus for determination of volatile oils. Add water through the top of reflux condenser until the graduated tube of B is filled and water overflows to flask A. Heat the flask gently in an electric heating jacket or by other suitable means. Heat to boiling, and remain for about 3 h, until the volume of oil does not increase any more. Stop heating, stand for a few minutes, and open the stopcock at the lower part of B, run off the water layer slowly until the oily layer is 5mm above the 0 sacle. Stand for at least 1h, open the stopcock again, run off the remaining water layer carefully until the oily layer is just on the 0 sacle. Read the volume of oil in the graduated portion of the tube and calculate the content of volatile oil, expressed as percentage (V/W) according to the following formula.

$$\text{Content of volatileoil}(\%) = \frac{\text{the volume of volatile oil(ml)}}{\text{the weight of the drug(g)}} \times 100\% \qquad (8-1)$$

Method B：Transfer 300ml of water and a few glass beads to flask A. Add water through the top of B until the graduated tube of B is filled and water overflows to flask A. Add 1ml of xylene with a pipette and then connect the reflux condenser C to B. Heat to boiling, continue to distill at a proper rate. Stop heating after 30min, stand for at least 15min. Read the volume of xylene in the graduated portion of the tube. Carry out the procedure described under Method A. Subtract the volume of xylene previously observed from the volume of the oily layer, the remainder is taken to be the content of volatile oil, expressed as percentage. The calculation formula is shown as follows.

$$\text{Content of volatile oil}(\%) = \frac{\text{the volume(the oily layer} - \text{xylene)(ml)}}{\text{the weight of the drug(g)}} \times 100\% \quad (8-2)$$

2. Determination of extractives

（1）Determination of water – soluble extractives

Cold maceration method：Weigh accurately 4g of the coarse powder of Morindae Officinalis

Radix to a 250ml stoppered conical flask, add accurately 100ml of water, and stopper tightly. Macerate the drug with shaking for 6 h and stand for 18h. Filter rapidly through a dry filter, transfer accurately 20ml of filtrate to an evaporating dish, previously dried to constant weight, evaporate to dryness on a water bath. Dry at 105℃ for 3h, allow to cool for 30min in a desiccator. Weigh rapidly and accurately, calculate the percentage of water – soluble extractives according to the following formula.

Hot maceration method: Weigh accurately 4g of the powered Dipsaci Radix to a 250ml stoppered conical flask, accurately add 100ml of water, stopper tightly and weigh, stand for 1h, connect flask A to condense. Heat to boiling, and remain boiling for 1h. Allow to cool, take off the flask, stopper tightly and weigh, replenish the loss of weight with water, shake well and filter through a dry filter. Transfer accurately 25ml of the filtrate to an evaporating dish, previously dried to constant weight, and evaporate to dryness on a water bath. Dry at 105℃ for 3h and allow to cool for 30min in a desiccator. Weigh rapidly and accurately, calculate the percentage of water – soluble extractives according to the following formula.

water or alcohol soluble extractives(%)

$$= \frac{(\text{weight of extrusion and evaporation pan} - \text{weight of evaporation pan}) \times \text{volume of water or alcohol}}{\text{weight of the sample} \times \text{volume of the filtrate}} \times 100\%$$

$$(8-3)$$

(2) Determination of alcohol – soluble extractives

The determination of alcohol – soluble extractives also includes hot maceration method and cold maceration method. The procedure is same as that of the water – soluble extractive except that the different concentration of ethanol or methanol is used as solvent instead of water.

Cold maceration method: Weighed accurately about 4 g of the powder of Forsythiae Fructus, carry out the determination of water – soluble extractives, cold maceration method, using 65% ethanol instead of water.

Hot maceration method: Weighed accurately about 4 g of the powder of Eucommiae Cortex, carry out the determination of water – soluble extractives, hot maceration method, using 75% ethanol instead of water.

(3) Determination of ether – soluble extractives

Weigh accurately about 2g of the powder of Angelicae Pubescentis Radix (through No. 4 sieve), store in phosphorus pentoxide desiccant for 48h. Place the powder in Soxhlet extractor. Add 70ml of sulfuric ether heating on a water bath under reflux for 4h, cool and filter, rinse the flask and extractor with a little volume of ether, combine the washings and filtrate into a 100ml volumetric flask, and dilute with ether to the volume, mix well. Transfer accurately 50ml of the filtrate to an evaporating dish, previously dried to constant weight. Evaporate the ether extraction to dryness on a water bath at low temperature, transfer the residue to the desiccator containing phosphorus pentoxide, store for 24h, take out the residue, weigh rapidly and accurately, calculate the content of ether – soluble extractives according to the following formula.

ether – soluble extractives（%）

$$= \frac{(\text{weight of extractives and evaporation pan before drying} - \text{weight of extractives and evaporation pan after drying})}{\text{weight of the sample}} \times 100\%$$

$$(8-4)$$

【Assignments】

Record the procedures for determination of the volatile oils and extractives in the crude drugs, and calculate the contents.

【Discussion】

During determining volatile oils，what arekey factors that affect the results?

实验九　生药重金属及有害元素测定

【实验目的】

1. 了解生药重金属及有害元素的测定原理与方法。
2. 掌握雄黄中可溶性砷及总砷的测定方法。

【实验指导】

生药中一类重要的外源性有害物质是重金属和有害元素，主要有铅（Pb）、镉（Cd）、汞（Hg）、铜（Cu）、砷（As）等。

重金属总量常用硫代乙酰胺或硫化钠比色法测定，有害元素砷的测定常用古蔡氏法或二乙基二硫代氨基甲酸银法。单个重金属和有害元素测定常用原子吸收光谱法（atomic absorption spectrophotometry，AAS）和电感耦合等离子体质谱法（inductivelycoupledplasma - massspectrometry，ICP - MS）。

硫代乙酰胺法适用于溶于水、稀酸或乙醇的药物中的重金属限量检查。检查原理为硫代乙酰胺在弱酸性（pH 值为 3.5 醋酸盐缓冲溶液）条件下水解，产生硫化氢，与重金属离子生成黄色到棕黑色的硫化物均质混悬液，与一定量标准铅溶液经同法处理后所呈颜色比较，判定供试品中重金属是否符合限量规定。

ASS 法的测定对象是呈原子状态的金属元素和部分非金属元素，如铅、镉、汞、铜、砷等，系由待测元素灯发出的特征谱线通过供试品经原子化产生原子蒸汽时，被蒸汽中待测元素的基态原子吸收，通过测定辐射光强度减弱的程度测定供试品中待测元素含量的一种光谱分析方法。

ICP - MS 法是将被测物质用电感耦合等离子体离子化后，按离子的质荷比分离，测量各种离子谱峰强度的一种分析方法。主要用于进行多种元素的同时测定，并可与其他色谱分离技术联用，进行元素形态及其价态分析。

【仪器及试剂】

1. 仪器

液相色谱 - 电感耦合等离子体质谱联用仪、离心管、微孔滤膜、超声波清洗器、锥形瓶等。

2. 试剂

蒸馏水、亚砷酸根溶液标准物质、砷酸根溶液标准物质、乙二胺四醋酸二钠、人工肠液、硫酸钾、硫酸铵、硫酸、酚酞指示液、40% 氢氧化钠溶液、碳酸氢钠、0.05mol/L 碘滴定液、淀粉指示液等。

【实验材料】

雄黄。

【实验步骤】

1. 测定雄黄中可溶性砷含量

（1）对照品贮备溶液的制备

分别精密量取亚砷酸根溶液标准物质、砷酸根溶液标准物质适量，加水制成每1ml含两种价态砷（均以砷计）各2μg的混合溶液。

（2）对照品标准曲线溶液的制备

精密吸取对照品贮备溶液适量，加0.02mol/L乙二胺四醋酸二钠溶液分别制成每1ml含两种价态砷各5、20、50、100、200、500、1000ng（均以砷计）的系列溶液。

（3）供试品溶液的制备

取本品粉末（过五号筛）约30mg，精密称定，置250ml塑料量瓶中，加人工肠液约200ml，摇匀，置37℃水浴中超声处理（功率300W，频率45kHz）2小时（每隔15分钟充分摇匀一次），放冷，用人工肠液稀释至刻度，摇匀，取适量置50ml塑料离心管中，静置20～24小时，用洗耳球轻轻吹去上层表面溶液，吸取中层溶液约15ml（吸取时应避免带入颗粒），用微孔滤膜（10μm）滤过，精密量取续滤液5ml，置50ml塑料量瓶中，加0.02mol/L乙二胺四醋酸二钠溶液稀释至刻度，摇匀。同法制备试剂空白溶液。

（4）测定法

分别精密吸取标准曲线溶液与供试品溶液各20μl，注入液相色谱－电感耦合等离子体质谱联用仪，测定。以标准曲线溶液测得不同价态砷的峰面积为纵坐标，相应浓度为横坐标，绘制标准曲线，计算供试品中可溶性砷（以三价砷和五价砷总量计）含量。

2. 测定雄黄中总砷含量

取雄黄粉末约0.1g，精密称定，置锥形瓶中，加硫酸钾1g、硫酸铵2g与硫酸8ml，用直火加热至溶液澄明，放冷，缓缓加水50ml，加热微沸3～5分钟，放冷，加酚酞指示液2滴，用40%氢氧化钠溶液中和至显微红色，放冷，用0.25mol/L硫酸溶液中和至褐色，加碳酸氢钠5g，摇匀后，用0.05mol/L的碘滴定液滴定，至近终点时，加淀粉指示液2ml，滴定至溶液显紫色。每1ml碘滴定液相当于5.348mg的二硫化二砷。计算供试品中总砷（以二硫化二砷计）含量。

【实验报告】

记录雄黄砷含量测定步骤，分别计算可溶性砷及总砷含量。

【思考题】

以雄黄中可溶性砷及总砷含量测定为例，怎样科学评价矿物性生药的安全性？

Experiment 9　Determination of Heavy Metal and Harmful Elements in Crude Drugs

【Objective】

1. To know the principle and method for determination of heavy metals and harmful elements in crude drugs.

2. To master the methods for determination of soluble arsenic and total arsenic in Realgar.

【Principle】

Heavy metals and harmful elements, mainly including lead (Pb), cadmium (Cd), mercury (Hg), copper(Cu), arsenic(As), reprent a class of exogenous harmful substances in crude drugs.

The total amount of heavy metals is usually determined by thioacetamide or sodium sulfide colorimetric reaction, and arsenic is usually determined by Gutzeitor silver diethyl dithiocarbamate method. Atomic absorption spectrometry(AAS) and inductively coupled plasma spectrometry(ICP – MS) are widely used for determination of single heavy metals and harmful elements.

Thioacetamide method is suitable forlimit test of heavy metals in water, dilute acid or ethanol soluble drugs. Its principle is that thioacetamide hydrolyses in acetate buffer solution(pH = 3.5), produces hydrogen sulfide, which reacts with heavy metal ions to produce yellow to dark brown suspension of sulfide. The color so produced is compared to the color produce similarly in a control containing an amount of standard lead solution, so as to justify whether the heavy metals in test samples meet the limit.

ASS method can be used to determine metal elements in the atomic state and some non – metallic elements, such as lead, cadmium, mercury, copper, arsenic, etc. Its principle is that when the characteristic spectral line emitted from the lamp of test edelement passes through atomic vapor generated by atomization of test sample, it is absorbed by the ground – state atom, then the element to be tested can be determined by measurement of the weakened radiation intensity.

ICP – MS method is an analytical method to measure the strength of various ion spectral peaks after the substances are ionized by inductively coupled plasma and separated according to the mass charge ratio of ions. It can be used for simultaneous determincation of several elements. After coupled to other chromatographic techniques, it also can be used for analysis of elemental forms and valence states.

【Materials】

Realgar.

【Instruments and reagents】

1. Instruments

Liquid chromatography – inductively coupled plasma mass spectrometry (LC – ICPMS), Eppendorf tube, microporous filter membrane, ultrasonic cleaner, plastic volumetric flask, plastic centrifuge tube, conical flask.

2. Reagents

Distilled water, arsenite acid standard solution, arsenate acid standard solution, ethylenediamine tetraacetic acid disodium, artificial intestinal liquid, potassium sulfate, ammonium sulfate, sulfuric acid, phenolphthalein IS, 40% sodium hydroxide, sodium bicarbonate, 0.05mol/L of iodine VS, starch IS.

【Experimental Procedures】

1. Determination of soluble arsenic

(1) Preparation of stocking solution of reference substances

Accurately measure appropriate volume of arsenicus acid standard solution and arsenic acid standard solution add water to produce a mixed solution containing two kinds of valence state arsenic (both calculated as arsenic) 2μg per ml, as the stocking solution.

(2) Preparation of calibration solutions of reference substances

Accurately measure appropriate volume of the stocking solution, add 0.02mol/L ethylenediamine tetraacetic acid disodium solution to produce a series of calibration solutions containing two kinds of valence state arsenic(both calculated as arsenic) 5, 20, 50, 100, 200, 500, and 1000 ng per ml, as the calibration solutions.

(3) Preparation of test solution

Weigh accurelately about 30mg of Realgar powder(through No. 5 sieve) to a 250ml plastic volumetric flask, add about 200ml artificial intestinal liquid, shake well, ultrasonicate on a 37℃ water bath for 2h(shake violently every 15min), allow to cool, dilute to volume with artificial intestinal liquid, shake well. Measure appropriate volume of diluent to a 50ml plastic centrifuge tube, stand for 20 to 24h, gently blow off the upper surface solution with arubber suction bulb, measure about 15ml of the middle layer solution, filter with microporous membrane (10μm). Measure accurately the subsequent filtrate to a 50ml plastic volumetric flask, add 0.02mol/L ethylenediamine tetraacetic acid disodium sodium solution to volume, shakewell. Prepare the blank solution as above described.

(4) Assay

Accurately inject 20μl of each of calibration solution and test solution, respectively, into the column of HPLC – ICP MS, record peak areas. Plot the calibration curve, using the peak area of different valence arsenic measured as ordinate and corresponding concentration as abscissa, calculate the content of soluble arsenic, calculated as the sum of trivalent arsenic and pentavalent arsenic.

2. Determination of total arsenic

Accurately weight 0.1g of the powder of Realgar in a 250ml conical flask with 1g of potassium sulfate, 2g of ammonium sulfate and 8ml of sulfuric acid until the solution becomes clear. Allow to cool, add 50ml of water slowly, heat to boil gently for 3 ~ 5min and allow to cool. Add 2 drops of phenolphthalein IS, neutralize with 40% of sodium hydroxide solution until it becomes pale red, allow to cool, neutralize with 0. 25mol/L of sulfuric acid solutuion to colourless. Add 5g of sodium bicarbonate, shake well, titrate with 0. 05mol/L of iodine volumetric solution, towards the end of titration, add 2ml of starch indicator solution, continue to titrate until a purplish – blue color is produced. Each ml of iodine volumetric solution is equivalent to 5. 348mg of arsenic disulfide. Calculate the content of total arsenic, calculated as arsenic disulfide.

【Assignments】

Record the procedures for determination of arsenic in Realgar, calculate the contents of soluble arsenic and total arsenic, respectively.

【Discussion】

How to scientifically evaluate the safety of mineral crude drugs, using Realgar as a case?

实验十　农药残留量测定

【实验目的】

了解生药农药残留量测定方法。

【实验指导】

生药在种植、采收、包装运输、贮藏等各个环节都有可能和农药接触而受到污染。残留农药包括有机氯农药、有机磷农药和拟除虫菊酯类农药等。残留农药的测定方法主要有气相色谱法、气相色谱－质谱联用法、柱后衍生－高效液相色谱法、液相色谱－质谱联用法等。

【仪器及试剂】

1. 仪器

气相色谱仪、10ml 量瓶、100ml 具塞锥形瓶、旋转蒸发仪等。

2. 试剂

石油醚、丙酮、无水硫酸钠、弗罗里硅土、微晶纤维素、氧化铝、乙醚、氯氰菊酯标准品、氰戊菊酯标准品、溴氰菊酯标准品等。

【实验材料】

桔梗。

【实验步骤】

1. 色谱条件与系统适用性试验

以（5%苯基）甲基聚硅氧烷为固定液的弹性石英毛细管柱（30m × 0.32mm × 0.25μm），^{63}Ni – ECD 电子捕获检测器。进样口温度270℃，检测器温度330℃。不分流进样。程序升温：初始160℃，保持 1 分钟，每分钟 10℃升至278℃，保持 0.5 分钟，每分钟 1℃升至290℃，保持 5 分钟。理论板数按溴氰菊酯峰计算应不低于 10^5，两个相邻色谱峰的分离度应大于1.5。

2. 对照品贮备溶液的制备

精密称取氯氰菊酯、氰戊菊酯及溴氰菊酯农药对照品适量，用石油醚（60～90℃）分别制成每1ml 含20～25μg 的溶液，即得。

3. 混合对照品贮备溶液的制备

精密量取上述各对照品贮备液 1ml，置 10ml 量瓶中，用石油醚（60～90℃）稀释至刻度，摇匀，即得。

4. 混合对照品工作溶液的制备

精密量取上述混合对照品贮备液，用石油醚（60～90℃）制成每1L分别含0、2、8、40、200μg 的溶液，即得。

5. 供试品溶液的制备

取桔梗供试品，粉碎成粉末（过三号筛），取约 1 ~ 2g，精密称定，置 100ml 具塞锥形瓶中，加石油醚（60 ~ 90℃）–丙酮（4 : 1）混合溶液 30ml，超声处理 15 分钟，滤过，药渣再重复上述操作 2 次后，合并滤液，滤液用适量无水硫酸钠脱水后，于 40 ~ 45℃减压浓缩至近干，用少量石油醚（60 ~ 90℃）多次溶解并蒸干至丙酮除净，残渣用适量石油醚（60 ~ 90℃）溶解，置混合小柱〔从上至下依次为无水硫酸钠 2g、弗罗里硅土 4g、微晶纤维素 1g、氧化铝 1g、无水硫酸钠 2g，用石油醚（60 ~ 90℃）–乙醚（4 : 1）混合溶液 20ml 预洗〕上，用石油醚（60 ~ 90℃）–乙醚（4 : 1）混合溶液 90ml 洗脱，收集洗脱液，于 40 ~ 45℃减压浓缩至近干，再用石油醚（60 ~ 90℃）3 ~ 4ml 重复操作至乙醚除净，用石油醚（60 ~ 90℃）溶解并转移至 5ml 量瓶中，并稀释至刻度，摇匀，即得。

6. 测定法

分别精密吸取供试品溶液和与之相对应浓度的混合对照品工作溶液各 1μl，注入气相色谱仪，按外标法计算供试品中三种拟除虫菊酯农药残留量。

【实验报告】

记录桔梗拟除虫菊酯农药残留量测定的步骤，并计算三种拟除虫菊酯农药残留量。

【思考题】

常用的气相色谱检测器有哪些？各自适用于何种待测物的检测？

Experiment 10　Determination of Pesticide Residues in Crude Drugs

【Objective】

To know the method for determination of pesticide residues in crude drugs.

【Principle】

Crude drugs may be contaminated by pesticides invarious processes, such as planting, harvesting, packaging, transportation, and storage. The type of pesticide residues in crude drugs includes organochlorine pesticides, organophosphorus pesticides and pyrethroid pesticides. For determination of pesticide residues, there are several methods including gas chromatography, gas chromatography – mass spectrometry, pre – column derivatization high performance liquid chromatography, and liquid chromatography – mass spectrometry, etc..

【Instruments and reagents】

1. Instruments

Gas chromatograph, 10ml volumetric flask, 100ml stoppered conical flask, rotary evaporator.

2. Reagents

Petroleum ether, acetone, anhydrous sodium sulfate, Flori silica, microcrystalline cellulose, alumina, ether, cypermethrin reference substance, fenvaleratereference substance, deltamethrin reference substance.

【Materials】

Platycodonis Radix.

【Experimental Procedures】

1. Chromatographic system and system suitability

Column: an elastic quartz capillary column (30m × 0.32mm × 0.25μm) with (5% phenyl) methyl polysiloxane as the stationary liquid; detector: ^{63}Ni – ECD electron capture detector. Injector temperature: 270℃; Detector temperature: 330℃. Splitless injection. Programmed temperature: initial tempearature 160℃, maintaining for 1min, increasing at 10℃ per min to 278℃, maintaining for 0.5min, increasing at 1℃ per min to 290℃, maintaining for 5min. Number of theoretical plates of the column: not less than 10^5, calculated with reference to the peak of deltamethrin. Resolution of two adjacent chromatographic peaks: more than 1.5.

2. Preparation of stocking solution of reference substances

Accurately measure appropriate volume of cypermethrin, fenvalerate and deltamethrin pesticide reference substances, and dilute with petroleum ether (60～90℃) to produce a solution containing about 20～25μg per ml, as stocking solution.

3. Preparation of mixed stocking solution of reference substances

Accurately measure 1ml of each of the above – mentioned stocking solutions to a 10ml volemetric flask, dilute with petroleum ether (60～90℃) to volume, shake well.

4. Preparation of mixed working solutions of reference substances

Accurately measure each of the above – mentioned mixed stocking solution, dilute withpetroleum ether (60～90℃) to produce a series of working solutions containing 0,2,8,40, and 200μg per ml, respectively.

5. Preparation of test solution

Weigh accurately about 1～2g of Platycodonis Radix powder (through No. 3 sieve) to a 100ml stoppered conical flask with, add 30ml of a mixture of petroleum ether (60～90℃) and acetone (4:1), ultrasonicate for 15min, filter. Repeat the above mentioned extraction procedure twice, combine the filtrate, dehydrate with an appropriate amount of anhydrous sodium sulfate, and concentrate under reduced pressure at 40～45℃ to near dryness. Repeat the dissolvation – evaporation procedure with a small amount of petroleum ether (60～90℃) until the acetone is completely removed. Dissolve the residue with an appropriate amount of petroleum ether (60～90℃), load on a mixing column (packed from top to bottom with anhydrous sodium sulfate 2g, Flori silica 4g, microcrystalline cellulose 1g, alumina 1g, anhydrous sodium sulfate 2g., Pre – wash the column with 20ml of a mixture of petroleum ether (60～90℃) anddiethyl ether (4:1), then elute with 90ml of a mixture of petroleum ether (60～90℃) and diethyl ether (4:1), collect the eluate, concentrate under reduced pressure at 40～45℃ to near dryness. Repeat the dissolvation – evaporation procedure with 3～4ml of petroleum ether (60～90℃) until ether is completely removed. Dissolve the residuein petroleum ether(60~90℃), and transfer to a 5ml of volemetric flask, dilute to volume, shake well.

6. Assay

Accurately measure each of testsolution and mixed working solution with corresponding concentration 1μl, respectively, inject into the gas chromatograph, and calculate the contents of three pyrethroid pesticide residues, according to external standard method.

【Assignments】

Record the procedures for determination of pesticide residues in Platycodonis Radix, calculate their contents.

【Discussion】

What detectors coupled to gas chromatography are there? What kind of analytes are they applicable to?

第二篇　验证性实验

Chapter Two　Confirmatory Experiments

实验十一　菌类生药——灵芝、茯苓

【实验目的】

1. 掌握灵芝和茯苓主要的性状及显微鉴别特征。
2. 熟悉鉴定灵芝和茯苓的方法。

【实验指导】

菌类生药由菌丝构成，显微特征包括菌丝团、菌丝、孢子等。主要化学成分为多糖类、氨基酸类、生物碱类、甾醇类和萜类等。常见生药包括冬虫夏草、灵芝、茯苓等。

灵芝为多孔菌科真菌赤芝 *Ganoderma lucidum*（Leyss. ex Fr.）Karst. 或紫芝 *Ganoderma sinensis* Zhao，Xu et Zhang 的干燥子实体。

茯苓为多孔菌科真菌茯苓 *Poriacocos*（Schw.）Wolf 的干燥菌核。

【仪器与试剂】

1. 仪器

光学显微镜、酒精灯、解剖针、载玻片、盖玻片等。

2. 试剂

水合氯醛溶液、斯氏液、稀甘油、蒸馏水等。

【实验材料】

灵芝（赤芝或紫芝）的药材标本及粉末；茯苓药材标本及粉末。

【实验步骤】

1. 性状鉴别

（1）灵芝

①赤芝：外形呈伞状，菌盖肾形、半圆形或近圆形，直径 10～18cm，厚 1～2cm。皮壳坚硬，黄褐色至红褐色，有光泽，具环状棱纹和辐射状皱纹，边缘薄而平截，常稍内卷。菌肉白色至淡棕色。菌柄圆柱形，侧生，少偏生，长 7～15cm，直径 1～3.5cm，红褐色至紫褐色，光亮。孢子细小，黄褐色。气微香，味苦涩。

②紫芝：皮壳紫黑色，有漆样光泽。菌肉锈褐色。菌柄长 17～23cm（图 11 - 1）。

③栽培品：子实体较粗壮、肥厚，直径 12～22cm，厚 1.5～4cm。皮壳外常被有大量粉尘样的黄褐色孢子。

（2）茯苓

①茯苓个：呈类球形、椭圆形或不规则团块，大小不一。外皮薄而粗糙，棕褐色或黑褐色，具皱缩纹理，有时部分剥落。质坚实，破碎面颗粒性，近边缘淡红色，有细小蜂窝样孔洞，内部白色，少数粉红色，有的中间抱有松根。气微，味淡，嚼之粘牙。

②茯苓块：呈立方块状或方块状厚片，大小不一，白色、淡红色或淡棕色（图 11 -2）。

③茯苓片：呈不规则厚片，厚薄不一。白色、淡红色或淡棕色，平滑细腻。

2. 显微鉴别

（1）灵芝

粉末浅棕色、棕褐色至紫褐色。菌丝散在或黏结成团，无色或淡棕色，细长，稍弯曲，有分枝，直径 2.5～6.5μm。孢子褐色，卵形，顶端平截，外壁无色，内壁有疣状突起，长 8～12μm，宽 5～8μm（图 11 -3）。

（2）茯苓

粉末用斯氏液装片，可见无色不规则形颗粒团块、末端钝圆的分枝状团块及细长菌丝；遇水合氯醛溶液黏化成胶冻状，加热团块物深化。用5%氢氧化钾溶液装片，可见菌丝细长，稍弯曲，有分支，无色（内层菌丝）或带棕色（外层菌丝），长短不一，直径 3～8（～16）μm，横隔偶见（图 11 -4）。

【实验报告】

1. 记述灵芝药材性状，记述茯苓药材性状，包括茯苓个、茯苓皮、茯苓块。
2. 绘灵芝粉末特征图，绘茯苓粉末特征图，示菌丝及多糖团块。

【思考题】

怎样检测破壁灵芝孢子粉的破壁率?

Experiment 11　Identification of Ganoderma and Poria(Fungi)

【Objective】

1. To master the Macroscopic and microscopic identification of Ganoderma and Poria.
2. To be familiar with the method of determination of Ganoderma and Poria.

【Principle】

The microscopic characteristics of the crude drug from Fungi: hypha ball, hypa and spore. The main constituents in the crude drug are polysaccharides, amino acids, alkaloids, sterols, terpenoids and so on. The important drugs from fungi contains Cordyceps, Ganoderma and Poria.

Ganoderma is the dried fruiting body of *Ganoderma lucidum* (Leyss. ex Fr.) Karst. or *G.*

sinensis Zhao, Xu et Zhang(Family Polyporaceae).

Poria is the dried sclerotium of *Poria*cocos(Schw.) Wolf(Family Polyporaceae).

【Instruments and Reagents】

1. Instruments

Optical microscope, alcohol lamp, anatomical needle, slide, cover glass.

2. Reagents

Chloral hydrate solution, glycerin – acetic acid solution, dilute glycerin, distilled water.

【Materials】

Referencecrude drug of Ganoderma and its powders; Reference crude drug of Poria and its powder.

【Experimental Procedures】

1. Macroscopic identification

(1)Ganoderma

①*Ganoderma lucidum*: Outline fimbriae, pileus reunion. semi – rounded or surrounded, 10 ~ 18cm in diameter, 1 ~ – 2cm thick. Shell hard, yellowish – brown to reddish – brown, lustrous, with circular arrested stripe and radiate wrinkle, edge thin and even, frequently incurved slightly. The inner part white to brownish. Strip saturated chamber, laterally grown, few leanings grown, 7 ~ 15cm long, 1 ~ 3. 5cm in diameter. reddish – brown to purplish brown, luminous Spore small and fine, yellowish – brown. Odour, slightly aromatic, taste, bitter and puckery.

②*G. sinensis*: Shell purplish – black, with lacquer – like luster. Sporophore rusty – brown. Strip 17 ~ 23cm long.

③Cultivated Ganoderma: Sporophore relatively sturdy, plump, 1 ~ 22cm in diameter. 1. 5 ~ 4cm thick. Shell frequently coated with a large of yellowish – brown powder – like spores.

(2)Poria

①Fulingge: Subglobose, ellipsoid or irregular – shaped, variable in size. The outer skin thin and rough, brown to blackish – brown, conspicuously shriveled and striated, sometimes partly dropped off. Texture hard and compact, fracture granular, near the edge pale red, with smart honeycombing hollows, inner part white, rarely reddish, some showing the penetrating roots of pine in the center. Odour, slight, taste, weak and sticky when chewed.

②Fulingpi (pared skin of Poria): Irregular pieces, externally brown to blackish – brown, internally white or pale brown, texture relatively loose and soft, slightly elastic.

③Fulingkuai(peeled and sliced Poria): Occurring in pieces or slices, white, pale red or pale brown.

2. Microscopic Identification

(1)Powder of Ganoderma

Hyphae scattered or grouped, colorless or pale brown, slim, slightly curved, branched, 2. 5 ~ 6. 5μm in diameter.

Spores brown, ovate, apex even, external walls colorless, inner walls with protuberance. 8 ~ 12μm long, 5 ~ 8μm wide.

(2) Powder of Poria

Slides with glycerol – acetic acid TS: irregular granular masses, branched masses and slender hyphae colorless; dissolved gradually on mounting in chloral hydrate solution, the masses dissolved on heating.

Slides with 5% potassium hydroxide solution: hyphae slender, slightly curved, branched, colorless (inner hyphae) or pale brown (outer hyphae), uneven in size, 3 ~ 8μm (rarely up to 16μm) in diameter, trabecula occasionally seen.

【Assignments】

1. Describe the description of Ganoderma and Poria examined, including Fulingge, Fulingpi, Fulingkuai.

2. Draw the characteristic drawing of the powder of Ganoderma andPoria, showing hyphae and polysaccharide masses.

【Discussion】

How to determine the wall – broken rate of spore from powdered Ganoderma?

实验十二　裸子植物类生药——麻黄

【实验目的】

1. 掌握麻黄类生药的性状及显微主要鉴别特征。
2. 了解裸子植物生药的主要鉴别特征。

【实验指导】

裸子植物茎的维管束环状排列，具有形成层，次生木质部大多为管胞，极少有导管；韧皮部中有筛胞而无伴胞。该类生药主要含有黄酮类、生物碱类、树脂及挥发油类等成分。代表生药包括银杏叶、红豆杉、麻黄等。

麻黄为麻黄科植物草麻黄 *Ephedra sinica* Stapf、中麻黄 *E. intermedia* Schrenk et C. A. Mey. 或木贼麻黄 *E. equisetina* Bge. 的干燥草质茎。

【仪器与试剂】

1. 仪器
光学显微镜、酒精灯、解剖针、载玻片、盖玻片等。

2. 试剂
水合氯醛溶液、稀甘油、蒸馏水等。

【实验材料】

麻黄（草麻黄、中麻黄或木贼麻黄）药材标本及粉末；麻黄茎横切面永久制片。

【实验步骤】

1. 性状鉴别

（1）草麻黄

细长圆柱形，少分支，直径 1~2mm，有时带少量灰棕色木质茎。表面淡绿色至黄绿色，有细纵棱，触之微有粗糙感，节明显，节间长 2~6cm，节上有膜质鳞叶，红棕色，长 3~4mm，裂片 2 裂（稀 3 裂），裂片锐三角形，先端灰白色，反曲基部联合成筒状。体轻，质脆，断面类圆形或扁圆形，略呈纤维性，中心暗红棕色。气微香，味涩、微苦。

（2）中麻黄

分枝较多，直径 1.5~3mm，有粗糙感。膜质鳞叶长 2~3mm，裂片 3（稀 2）；断面髓部呈三角状圆形。

（3）木贼麻黄

分枝较多，直径 1~1.5mm，无粗糙感。节间长 1.5~3cm，膜质鳞叶长 1~2mm，裂片 2（稀 3），上部短三角形，灰白色，先端多不反曲，基部棕红色至棕黑色（图 12-1）。

2. 显微鉴别

（1）茎节间横切面

①草麻黄：边缘有波状细棱脊 18～20 条。表皮细胞类方形，外壁厚，被厚的角质层，两棱脊间有下陷气孔；在棱脊内侧有下皮纤维束。皮层宽，有少数纤维散在。中柱鞘纤维束新月形，位于韧皮部外侧。维管束外韧型，8～10 个，形成层环类圆形。木质部类三角形。髓薄壁细胞壁非木化，常含红棕色块状物，偶有环髓纤维。表皮细胞外壁、皮层细胞及纤维壁均可见草酸钙砂晶（图 12－2）。

②中麻黄：棱脊 18～28 个；维管束 12～15 个，形成层环类三角形；薄壁细胞壁微木化，环髓纤维多。

③木贼麻黄：棱脊 13～14 个；维管束 8～10 个，形成层环类圆形；薄壁细胞壁木化，无环髓纤维。

（2）草麻黄粉末

表皮细胞类长方形，外壁布满草酸钙砂晶，角质层厚达 18μm。气孔特异，长圆形，保卫细胞侧面观似电话筒状。皮层纤维长，直径 10～24μm，壁厚，有的木化，壁上布满砂晶，形成嵌晶纤维。棕色块多见，呈类圆形、方形（图 12－3）。

【实验报告】

1. 列表记述三种麻黄草质茎横切面的组织特征，并绘草麻黄茎的横切面简图。

2. 绘草麻黄粉末特征图，示气孔、嵌晶纤维和导管。

【思考题】

麻黄药材红棕色髓部习称为"玫瑰心"，是其品质评价的重要指标。怎样证明该评价指标的合理性？

Experiment 12　Identification of Ephedrae Herba(Gymnospermae)

【Objective】

1. To master the Macroscopic and microscopic identification of Ephedrae Herba.

2. To understand the main characteristics for identification of Gymnosperms.

【Principle】

The microscopic characteristics of stem of Gymnosperms plants: stem vascular bundles arrange in a ring, and cambium ring surrounded. Secondary xylem consists of plenty of tracheidand very few ducts. Phloem contains sieve cells. The main constituents in the crude drug are flavonoids, alkaloids, resins, volatile oils and so on. The important drugs from Gymnosperms contains Ginkgo Folium, Taxi Ramulus et Folium seu Cortex, and Ephedrae Herba.

Ephedrae Herba consis the dried stems of *Ephedra sinica* Stapf、*Ephedra intermedia* Schrenk et C. A. Mey. or *Ephedra equisetina* Bge.

【Instruments and Reagents】

1. Instruments

Optical microscope, alcohol lamp, anatomical needle, slide, cover glass.

2. Reagents

Chloral hydrate solution, dilute glycerin, distilled water.

【Materials】

Reference crude drug of Ephedrae Herba and its powder; slides of stem transverse sections of *E. sinica*.

【Experimental Procedures】

1. Macroscopic identification

（1）Stem of *E. sinica*

Slenderly cylindrical, 1 ~ 2mm in diameter. Some with a few greyish – brown woody stems. Externally pale green to yellowish – green, with fine longitudinal ridges. Nodes distinct, internode 2 ~ 6cm long. Scaly leaves on the nodes membranous, reddish – brown, 3 ~ 4mm long, with 2 lobes (rarely 3), acutely triangular, apex greyish – white, reversed, based tubular and reddish – brown in color. Texture light, fragile, fracture, surrounded or elliptical, slightly fibrous, reddish – brown center. Odour, slightly aromatic; taste, astringent and slightly bitter.

（2）Stem of *E. intermedia*

Frequently branched, 1. 3 ~ 3mm in diameter, rough, membranous scaly leaves 2 ~ 3mm long, with 3 lobes(rarely 2 lobes). Fracture showing a triangular rounded pith.

（3）Stem of *E. equisetina*

Frequently branched, 1 ~ 1. 5mm in diameter, unrough. Internode 1. 5 ~ 3cm long. Membranous scaly leaves 1 ~ 2mm long, with 2 lobes (rarely 3 lobes), short – triangular, greyish – white, apex infrequently reversed, base brownish – red to brownish – black.

2. Microscopic identification

（1）Transverse section

①Stem of *E. sinica*: Waved – shaped fine ridges on fringe 18 ~ 20. Epidermal cells subsquare, covered with thick cuticle, sunken stomata located between two ridges. Hypodermal fiber bundles located in ridges. Cortex broad, a few fiber bundles scattered. Pericycle Fiber bundles crescent, outside of phloem. Collateral vascular bundles 8 ~ 10, cambium ring subrounded. Xylem subtriangular. Pithparenchymatous cells non – lignified, containing reddish – brown masses; occasionally showing perimedullary fibers. Outer wall of epidermal cells, cortex parenchymatous cells and fibers occurring sandy crystals of calcium oxalate.

②Stem of *E. intermedia*: Ridges 18 ~ 28; vascular bundles 12 ~ 15, cambium ring subtriangular. Pith parenchymatous cells slightly lignified, with numerous perimedullary fibers.

③Stem of *E. equisetina*: Ridges 13 ~ 14; vascular bundles 8 ~ 10, cambium ring subround. Pith parenchymatous lignified, without perimedullary fibers.

（2）Powder

Epidermal cells subsquare, outer wall covered with sandy crystals of calcium oxalate, cuticle up to 18μm thick. Special stoma, long – rounded, phone – like guard cells in side view. Cortical fibers slender, 10 ~ 24μm in diameter; thickened – walls, sometimes lignified, scattered with many sandy crystals, formed chimeric fibers. Brown lumps are square or rounded.

【Assignments】

1. Make a schedule to record the characters of transverse section of herbaceous stem of three species of Ephedrae Herba, and make a diagrammatic drawing of transverse section of stem of *E. sinica*.

2. Make a diagram of the characters of powder of Ephedrae Herba, and signify the stomata, chimeric fiber and vessel.

【Discussion】

The term of "Rose Heart" refers to the brownish – red pith of Ephedrae Herba, and it is traditionally used to evaluate the quality of this crude drug. How to demonstrate the rationality of this quality indicator?

实验十三　蓼科生药——大黄、何首乌

【实验目的】

1. 掌握大黄的性状及显微鉴别特征。
2. 掌握何首乌的性状鉴别特征。

【实验指导】

蓼科植物常为草本或灌木，茎节常膨大、托叶鞘膜质包茎；花两性或单性异株；单被，花被3～6，花瓣状，宿存。主要化学成分为蒽醌类、黄酮类、鞣质及各种苷类。常见生药包括大黄、何首乌、虎杖等。

大黄为蓼科植物掌叶大黄 *Rheum palmatum* L.、唐古特大黄 *Rheum tanguticum* Maxim，ex Balf. 或药用大黄 *Rheum officinale* Baill. 的干燥根和根茎。

何首乌为蓼科植物何首乌 *Polygonum multiflorum* Thunb. 的干燥块根。

【仪器与试剂】

1. 仪器
光学显微镜、酒精灯、解剖针、载玻片、盖玻片等。

2. 试剂
水合氯醛溶液、稀甘油、蒸馏水等。

【实验材料】

大黄、何首乌的药材标本及粉末；大黄根茎（髓部）横切面永久制片；何首乌块根横切面永久制片。

【实验步骤】

1. 性状鉴别

（1）大黄

本品呈圆柱形、圆锥形、卵圆形或不规则块状，长3～17cm，直径3～10cm。除尽外皮者表面黄棕色或红棕色，有的可见类白色网状纹理及星点（异常维管束）散在，残留的外皮棕褐色，多具绳孔及粗皱纹。质坚实，有的中心稍松软，断面淡红棕色或黄棕色，显颗粒性；根茎髓部宽广，有星点环列或散在；根木部发达，具放射状纹理，形成层环明显，无星点。气清香，味苦而微涩，嚼之粘牙，有砂粒感（图13-1）。

（2）何首乌

本品呈团块状或不规则纺锤形，长6～15cm，直径4～12cm。表面红棕色或红褐色，皱缩不平，有浅沟，并有横长皮孔样突起和细根痕。体重，质坚实，不易折断，断面浅黄棕色或浅红棕色，显粉性，皮部有4～11个类圆形异型维管束环列，形成云锦状花纹，中央木部较大，有的呈木心。气微，味微苦而甘涩（图13-2）。

2. 显微鉴别

（1）大黄

①根茎横切面：木栓层与皮层大多已除去。韧皮部筛管群明显。形成层环明显。木质部射线较密，宽2～4列细胞，内含棕色物；导管径向稀疏排列。髓部宽广，其中常见黏液腔，内有红棕色物；异型维管束散在，形成层类圆形，木质部在外，韧皮部在内，射线星芒状。薄壁细胞含草酸钙簇晶，并含多数淀粉粒（图13-3、13-4）。

②粉末：黄棕色。草酸钙簇晶，直径20～160μm，有的至190μm。网纹导管和具缘纹孔导管，非木化。淀粉粒较多，单粒类球形或多角形，直径3～44μm，脐点星状；复粒由2～8分粒组成（图13-5）。

（2）何首乌

①横切面：木栓层为数列细胞，充满棕色物。韧皮部较宽，散有类圆形异型维管束4～11个，为外韧型，导管稀少。根的中央形成层成环；木质部导管较少，周围有管胞和少数木纤维。薄壁细胞含草酸钙簇晶和淀粉粒（图13-6）。

②粉末：黄棕色。淀粉粒单粒类圆形，直径4～50μm，脐点人字形、星状或三叉状，大粒者隐约可见层纹；复粒由2～9分粒组成。草酸钙簇晶直径10～80（160）μm，偶见簇晶与较大的方形结晶合生。棕色细胞类圆形或椭圆形，壁稍厚，胞腔内充满淡黄棕色、棕色或红棕色物质，并含淀粉粒。具缘纹孔导管直径17～178μm 棕色块散在，形状、大小及颜色深浅不一（图13-7）。

【实验报告】

1. 绘大黄根茎髓部异型维管束简图。
2. 绘何首乌横切面简图。

【思考题】

1. 何首乌的"云锦样花纹"是什么组织构造？
2. 除大黄外，还有哪些生药具有异型维管束？在构造上有何不同？

Experiment 13　Identification of Rhei Radix et Rhizoma and Polygoni Multiflori Radix(Polygonaceae)

【Objective】

1. To master the macroscopic and microscopic identification of Rhei Radix et Rhizoma.

2. To master the macroscopic identification of Polygoni Multiflori Radix.

【Principle】

Polygonaceae crude drugs are often herbs or shrubs, stems often swollen nodes, ostitium sheath membranous phimosis and flowers bisexual or unisexual; perianth simple, perianth 3～6, petalate, persistent. The main chemical constituents are anthraquinones, flavonoids, tannins and various glycosides. The representative drugs from polygonaceae contain Rhei Radix et Rhizoma, Polygoni Multiflori Radix, Polygoni Cuspidati Rhizoma et Radix and so on.

Rhei Radix et Rhizoma are the dried roots and rhizomes of the Polygonaceae plants of *Rheum palmatum* L. , *Rheum tanguticum* Maxim, ex Balf. , or *Rheum officinale* Baill.

Polygoni Multiflori Radix is the dried tuberous root of the Polygonaceae plants of *Polygonum multiflorum* Thunb.

【Instruments and Reagents】

1. Instruments

Optical microscope, alcohol lamp, anatomical needle, slide, cover glass.

2. Reagents

Chloral hydrate solution, dilute glycerin, distilled water.

【Materials】

Reference crude drug of Rhei Radix et Rhizoma and its powder, reference crude drug of Polygoni Multiflori Radix and its powder; slides of rhizome (espiecally the pith) of *Rheum palmatum*; slides of root of *Polygonum multiflorum*.

【Experiment Procedures】

1. Macroscopic identification

(1) Rhei Radix et Rhizoma

In subcylindrical, conical, ovoid or irregular pieces. 3 ~ 17cm long, 3 ~ 10cm in diameter. Externally yellowish – brown to reddish – brown when peeled, sometimes whitish reticulations and scattered star spots (abnormal vascular bundles) visible, occasionally with brownish – black patches of cork, mostly with a hole through which the string passed, and coarse wrinkles. Texture compact, sometimes rather loose and soft in the center, fracture pale reddish – brown or yellowish – brown, granular. Pith of rhizome broad, with star spots arranged in a ring or irregularly scattered. Wood of the root well developed, lined radially, cambium ring distinct, without star spots. Odour, delicately aromatic; taste bitter and slightly astringent, sticky and gritty on chewing.

(2) Polygoni Multiflori Radix

Mass or irregular fusiform, 6 ~ 15cm long, 4 ~ 12cm in diameter. Externally reddish – brown, shrunken and uneven, shallowly grooved, with transverse elongated lenticel – like protrusions and fine rootlet scars. Texture heavy, compact, uneasily broken, fracture pale yellowish – brown or reddish – brown, starchy, bark exhibiting. 4 ~ 11 subrounded rings of abnormal vascular bundles, forming brocaded patterns, wood in central part relatively large, some having a woody core. Odour, slight; taste, bitterish, sweetish and astringent.

2. Microscopic Identification

(1) Rhei Radix et Rhizoma

①Transverse section: Most cork and phelloderm of root removed. In phloem, sieve tube groups in phloem distinct, parenchyma well developed. Cambium in a ring. Xylem with relatively dense rays, 2 – 4 cells wide, containing brown masses in ray cells, vessels loosely arrange radically. Pith broad, usually showing mucilage cavities, containing reddish – brown masses; abnormal vascular bundles scattered, cambium subrounded, xylem at the outside and phloem at the inside, rays stellately radiated. Parenchymatous cells containing clusters of calcium oxalate and abundant starch granules.

②Powder: Yellowish – brown. Clusters of calcium oxalate, 20 ~ 160μm, sometimes up to 190μm in diameter; Reticulated and bordered pitted vessels, unlignified. Starch grains fairly abundant, single granules subspheroidal or polygonal, 3 ~ 44μm in diameter, hilum stellate; compound granules consisting of 2 ~ 8 components.

(2) Polygoni Multiflori Radix

①Transverse section: Cork consisting of several layers of cells, filled with brown contents. Phloem relatively broad, scattered with 4 – 11 subrounded abnormal vascular bundles of collateral type, vessels rare. In the central part of a root cambium in a ring; vessels in xylem less, surrounded by some tracheids and a few xylem fibers. Parenchymatous cells containing starch granules, and clusters of calcium oxalate.

②Powder: Yellowish – brown. Simple starch granules subrounded, 4 ~ 50μm in diameter, hilum V – shaped, stellate or Y – shaped, striations of large ones fairly distinct; compound granules of 2 ~ 9 components. Clusters of calcium oxalate 10 ~ 80(160)μm in diameter, and clusters jointed with prisms occasionally found. Brown cells subrounded or elliptical, walls slightly thickened, lumina filled with yellowish – brown, brown or reddish – brown contents, and containing starch granules; bordered pitted vessels 17 – 178μm in diameter. Brown masses scattered, varying in shape, size and color.

【Assignments】

1. Make a diagnostic of transverse section of a star spot of Rhei Radix et Rhizoma.
2. Make a diagnostic of transverse section of Polygoni Multiflori Radix.

【Discussion】

1. What tissue stractures are the brocade patterns of Polygoni Multiflori Radix according to?
2. Do you know which tissues of crude drugs possess abnormal vascular bundles besides Rhei Radix et Rhizoma? What's the difference on the structure?

实验十四 苋科生药——牛膝、川牛膝

【实验目的】

1. 掌握牛膝及川牛膝的性状、显微鉴别特征。
2. 熟悉苋科植物根的主要鉴别特征。

【实验指导】

苋科植物多为草本，单叶互生，无托叶；花多两性，排成穗状、圆锥状或头状聚伞花序；单被，花被片3~5，干膜质；每朵花下常有1干膜质苞片及2小苞片。果为胞果，胚弯生。代表性生药有牛膝、川牛膝、青葙子等。

牛膝为苋科植物牛膝 *Achyranthes bidentata* Bl. 的干燥根。

川牛膝为苋科植物川牛膝 *Cyathula officinalis* Kuan 的干燥根。

【仪器与试剂】

1. 仪器

酒精灯、解剖针、载玻片、盖玻片等。

2. 试剂

水合氯醛溶液、稀甘油、蒸馏水等。

【实验材料】

牛膝药材标本及横切面永久切片；川牛膝药材标本、粉末及根横切面永久切片。

【实验步骤】

1. 性状鉴别

（1）牛膝

本品呈细长圆柱形，挺直或稍弯曲，长15~70cm，直径0.4~1cm。表面灰黄色或淡棕色，有微扭曲的细纵皱纹、排列稀疏的侧根痕和横长皮孔样的突起。质硬脆，易折断，受潮后变软，断面平坦，淡棕色，略呈角质样而油润，中心维管束木质部较大，黄白色，其外周散有多数黄白色点状维管束，断续排列成2~4轮。气微，味微甜而稍苦涩（图14-1）。

（2）川牛膝

本品呈近圆柱形，微扭曲，向下略细或有少数分枝，长30~60cm，直径0.5~3cm。表面黄棕色或灰褐色，具纵皱纹、支根痕和多数横长的皮孔样突起。质韧，不易折断，断面浅黄色或棕黄色，维管束点状，排列成数轮同心环。气微，味甜（图14-2）。

2. 显微鉴别

（1）牛膝

横切面

木栓层为数列扁平细胞，切向延伸。栓内层较窄。异型维管束外韧型，断续排列成2~

67

4 轮，最外轮的维管束较小，有的仅 1 至数个导管，束间形成层几连接成环，向内维管束较大；木质部主要由导管及小的木纤维组成，根中心木质部集成 2 ~ 3 群。薄壁细胞含有草酸钙砂晶（图 14 - 3，图 14 - 4）。

（2）川牛膝

①横切面：木栓细胞数列。栓内层窄。中柱大，三生维管束外韧型，断续排列成 4 ~ 11 轮，内侧维管束的束内形成层可见；木质部导管多单个，常径向排列，木化；木纤维较发达，有的切向延伸或断续连接成环。中央次生构造维管系统常分成 2 ~ 9 束，有的根中心可见导管稀疏分布。薄壁细胞含草酸钙砂晶、方晶（图 14 - 5、图 14 - 6）。

②粉末：棕色。草酸钙砂晶、方晶散在，或充塞于薄壁细胞中。具缘纹孔导管直径 10 ~ 80μm，纹孔圆形或横向延长呈长圆形，互列，排列紧密，有的导管分子末端呈梭形。纤维长条形，弯曲，末端渐尖，直径 8 ~ 25μm，壁厚 3 ~ 5μm，纹孔呈单斜纹孔或人字形，也可见具缘纹孔，纹孔口交叉成十字形，孔沟明显，疏密不一（图 14 - 7）。

【实验报告】

描绘牛膝及川牛膝的粉末特征图。

【思考题】

如何鉴别牛膝和川牛膝？

Experiment 14   Identification of Achyranthis Bidentatae Radix and Cyathulae Radix(Amaranthaceae)

【Objective】

1. To master the macroscopic and microscopic identification of Achyranthis Bidentatae Radix and Cyathulae Radix.

2. To learn the characters of roots of crude drugs from Amaranthaceae.

【Principle】

Amaranthaceae plants are mostly herbs, simple alternate leaves, no stipules; flowers mostly bisexual, arranged in spikes, panicles, or head cymes; tepals 3 ~ 5, dry membranous; there are often 1 dry membranous bract and 2 bracteoles under each flower. Fruit is cytoskeletal, germinal curving. The representative crude drugs are Achyranthis Bidentatae Radix, Cyathulae Radix, Celosiae Semen and so on.

Achyranthis Bidentatae Radix is the dried root of *Achyranthes bidentata* Bl. of Amaranthaceae plants.

Cyathulae Radix is the dried root of *Cyathula officinalis* Kuan.

【Instruments and Reagents】

1. Instruments

Optical microscope, alcohol lamp, anatomical needle, slide, cover glass.

2. Reagents

Chloral hydrate solution, dilute glycerin, distilled water.

【Materials】

Reference crude drugs of Achyranthis Bidentatae Radix and Cyathulae Radix; powder of Cyathulae Radix; slides of root of *Achyranthes bidentata* and *Cyathula officinalis*.

【Experimental Procedures】

1. Macroscopic identification

(1) Achyranthis Bidentatae Radix

Slender cylindrical, straight or slightly curved, 15 ~ 70cm, 0.4 ~ 1cm in diameter. Externally greyish – yellow or pale brown, with slightly twisted and fine longitudinal wrinkles, transverse lenticel – like protrudings and sparse rootlet scars. Texture hard and fragile, easily broken, softened when moistened, fracture even, pale brown, slightly horny and oily. Xylem of vascular bundles in the centre relatively large, yellowish – white, the outside scattered with many spotted vascular bundles arranged in 2 – 4 whorls. Odour slight; taste slightly sweet, somewhat bitter and astringent.

(2) Cyathulae Radix

Subcylindrical, somewhat twisted, slightly tapering downward or less – branched, 30 ~ 60cm long, 0.5 ~ 3cm in diameter. Externally yellowish – brown or greyish – brown, with longitudinal wrinkles, rootlet scars and numerous transverse lenticel – like protrusions. Texture tenacious, uneasily broken, fracture pale yellow or brownish – yellow, showing dotted vascular bundles, arranged in several concentric circles. Odour slight; taste sweet.

2. Microscopic identification

(1) Achyranthis Bidentatae Radix

Transverse section

Cork consisting of several layers of flattened cells, tangentially elongated. Phelloderm relatively narrow. Heteotype vascular bundles collateral, interruptedly arranged in 2 ~ 4 whorls, relatively small in the outermost whorl, some only 1 to several vessels, camblum nearly in a ring, vascular bundles relatively large inward; xylem consisting of vessels and small xylem fibers, aggregated into 2 ~ 3 groups in the central. Parenchymatous cells containing sand crystals of calcium oxalate.

(2) Cyathulae Radix

①Transverse section: Cork consisting of several layers of cells. Phelloderm narrow. Vascular saturated chamber large, tertiary vascular bundles collateral, interruptedly arranged in 4 ~ 11 whorls, intrafascicular cambium at the inner side visible; vessels singly scattered in xylem, lignified, arranged radially; xylary fibers well developed, sometimes tangentially elongated or arranged in an interrupted ring, secondary vascular system usually separated into 2 ~ 9 strands at the central, sometimes sparsely scattered vessels visible in the centre of root. Parenchymatous cells containing sand crystals and prisms of calcium oxalate.

② Powder: Brown. Sand and prism crystals of calcium oxalate scattered or filled in parenchymatous cells. Bordered pitted vessels $10 \sim 80\mu m$ in diameter, pits rounded or elongated transversely, alternative closely arranged, some vessel elements fusiform at the end. Fibers slat – shaped, curved, tapering towards the end, $8 \sim 25\mu m$ in diameter, walls $3 \sim 5\mu m$ thick, pits simple oblique or V – shaped, sometimes showing bordered pits, pit apertures crisscross, pit – canals distinct, dense or sparse.

【Assignments】

Draw characteristic drawings of the powder of Achyranthis Bidentatae Radix and Cyathulae Radix.

【Discussion】

How to distinguish the Achyranthis Bidentatae Radix and Cyathulae Radix?

实验十五　木兰科生药——厚朴、五味子

【实验目的】

1. 掌握厚朴、五味子的性状及显微鉴别特征。
2. 熟悉鉴定厚朴和五味子的主要方法。

【实验指导】

木兰科植物为灌木或乔木。单叶互生；托叶大，早落，形成托叶痕。花多两性，花被3基数；雄蕊和雌蕊多数，螺旋状排列在延长的花托上。木兰科生药主要含有挥发油类、生物碱类、倍半萜内酯类和木脂素类成分。代表生药有厚朴、辛夷、五味子等。

厚朴为木兰科植物厚朴 *Magnolia officinalis* Rehd. et Wils. 或凹叶厚朴 *Magnolia officinalis* Rehd. et Wils. var. *biloba* Rehd. et Wils. 的干燥干皮、根皮及枝皮。

五味子为木兰科植物五味子 *Schisandra chinensis* (Turcz.) Baill. 的干燥成熟果实，习称"北五味子"。

【仪器与试剂】

1. 仪器

光学显微镜、酒精灯、解剖针、载玻片、盖玻片等。

2. 试剂

水合氯醛溶液、稀甘油、蒸馏水等。

【实验材料】

厚朴、五味子的药材标本及粉末；厚朴（干皮）横切面永久制片；五味子（果实）横切面永久制片。

【实验步骤】

1. 性状鉴别

（1）厚朴

①干皮：呈卷筒状或双卷筒状，长30~35cm，厚0.2~0.7cm，习称"筒朴"；近根部的干皮一端展开如喇叭口，长13~25cm，厚0.3~0.8cm，习称"靴筒朴"。外表面灰棕色或灰褐色，粗糙，有时呈鳞片状，较易剥落，有明显椭圆形皮孔和纵皱纹，刮去粗皮者显黄棕色。内表面紫棕色或深紫褐色，较平滑，具细密纵纹，划之显油痕。质坚硬，不易折断，断面颗粒性，外层灰棕色，内层紫褐色或棕色，有油性，有的可见多数小亮星。气香，味辛辣、微苦（图15-1）。

②根皮（根朴）：呈单筒状或不规则块片；有的弯曲似鸡肠，习称"鸡肠朴"。质硬，较易折断，断面纤维性（图15-1）。

71

③枝皮（枝朴）：呈单筒状，长 10～20cm，厚 0.1～0.2cm。质脆，易折断，断面纤维性（图 15－1）。

（2）五味子

本品呈不规则的球形或扁球形，直径 5～8mm。表面红色、紫红色或暗红色，皱缩，显油润；有的表面呈黑红色或出现"白霜"。果肉柔软，种子 1～2，肾形，表面棕黄色，有光泽，种皮薄而脆。果肉气微，味酸；种子破碎后，有香气，味辛、微苦（图 15－2）。

2. 显微鉴别

（1）厚朴

①干皮组织横切面：木栓层为 10 余列细胞；有的可见落皮层。皮层外侧有石细胞环带，内侧散有多数油细胞和石细胞群。韧皮部射线宽 1～3 列细胞；纤维多数个成束；亦有油细胞散在（图 15－3）。

②干皮粉末：木栓细胞壁菲薄而平直，常多层重叠。纤维甚多，直径 15～32μm，壁甚厚，有的呈波浪形或一边呈锯齿状，木化，孔沟不明显。油细胞椭圆形或类圆形，直径 50～85μm，含黄棕色油状物。石细胞类方形、椭圆形、卵圆形或不规则分枝状，直径 11～65μm，有时可见层纹（图 15－4）。

（2）五味子

①横切面：外果皮为 1 列方形或长方形细胞，壁稍厚，外被角质层，散有油细胞；中果皮薄壁细胞 10 余列，含淀粉粒，散有小型外韧型维管束；内果皮为 1 列小方形薄壁细胞。种皮最外层为 1 列径向延长的石细胞，壁厚，纹孔和孔沟细密；其下为数列类圆形、三角形或多角形石细胞，纹孔较大；石细胞层下为数列薄壁细胞，种脊部位有维管束；油细胞层为 1 列长方形细胞，含棕黄色油滴；再下为 3～5 列小形细胞；种皮内表皮为 1 列小细胞，壁稍厚，胚乳细胞含脂肪油滴及糊粉粒（图 15－5，图 15－6）。

②粉末：暗紫色。种皮表皮石细胞表面观呈多角形或长多角形，直径 18～50μm，壁厚，孔沟极细密，胞腔内含深棕色物；种皮内层石细胞呈多角形、类圆形或不规则形，直径约至 83μm，壁稍厚，纹孔较大；果皮表皮细胞表面观类多角形，垂周壁略呈连珠状增厚，表面有角质线纹；表皮中散有油细胞；中果皮细胞皱缩，含暗棕色物，并含淀粉粒（图 15－7）。

【实验报告】

1. 记述厚朴干皮横切面的组织特征，并绘厚朴皮横切面组织简图。

2. 绘厚朴粉末特征图。

3. 绘五味子果实横切面组织简图。

4. 绘五味子粉末特征图，示种皮石细胞、果皮表皮细胞。

【思考题】

1. 皮类生药主要是来自于植物的何种组织？

2. "南五味子"的来源是什么？从性状上如何区别"北五味子"和"南五味子"？

Experiment 15　Identification of Magnoliae Officinalis Cortex and Schisandrae Chinensis Fructus(Magnoliaceae)

【Objective】

1. To master the characters of macroscopic and microscopic identification of Magnoliae Officinalis Cortex and Schisandrae Fructus.

【Principle】

Magnoliaceae plants are shrubs or trees, alternate leaves; stipules large, caducous, forming stipules mark. Flowers bisexual, perianth 3 – cardinal; the stamens and pistils, spirally arranged on an extended receptacle. The main constituents in the crude drug are alkaloids, lignans, volatile oils and sesquiterpenoids. The important drugs from magnoliaceae contains Magnoliae Officinalis Cortex, Magnoliae Flos, Schisandrae Chinensis Fructus.

Magnoliae Officinalis Cortex is the dry bark, root bark and branch bark of *Magnolia officinalis* Rehd. et Wils. or *Magnolia officinalis* Rehd. et Wils. var. *biloba* Rehd. et Wils. of Magnoliaceae plants.

Schisandrae Chinensis Fructusis the dried ripe fruit of *Schisandra chinensis* (Turcz.) Baill (Family Schisandraceae), commonly known as " Bei Wuweizi" (*Schisandra chinensis* growing in North of China).

【Instruments and Reagents】

1. Instruments

Optical microscope, alcohol lamp, anatomical needle, slide, cover glass.

2. Reagents

Chloral hydrate, dilute glycerin, distilled water.

【Materials】

Reference crude drugs and powders of Magnoliae Officinalis Cortex and Schisandrae Chinensis Fructus; slides of stem bark transverse section of *Magnolia officinalis*; slides of fruit transverse section of *Schisandra chinensis*.

【Experimental Procedures】

1. Macroscopic identification

(1)Magnoliae Officinalis Cortex

①Stem bark: Quilled singly or double quilled, 30 ~ 35cm long, 2 ~ 7mm thick, commonly known as "Tongpo"; the stem bark near the root has one end expanding like the mouth of a bell,

73

13 ~ 25cm long, 3 ~ 8mm thick, commonly known as "Xuetongpo". Outer surface greyish – brown, rough, sometimes scaly, easily exfoliated, with distinct elliptical lenticels and longitudinal wrinkles, appearing yellowish – brown when the coarse bark peeled; inner surface purplish – brown, relatively smooth, with fine and dense longitudinal striations and exhibits an oily trace on scratching. Texture hard, uneasily broken, fracture granular, grayish – brown in the outer layer and purplish – brown or brown in the inner layer, oily, sometimes with numerous small bright spots visible. Odour aromatic; taste pungent and slightly bitter.

②Root bark (Genpo): Quilled singly or pieced irregularly, some curved like chicken intestines, commonly known as "Jichangpo". Texture hard, easily broken, fracture fibrous.

③Branch bark(Zhipo): Quilled singly, 10 ~ 20cm long, 1 ~ 2mm thick. Texture fragile, easily broken, fracture fibrous.

(2)Schisandrae Chinensis Fructus

Irregularly spheroidal or compressed – spheroidal, 5 ~ 8mm in diameter. Externally red, purplish – red or dull red, shrunken, oily, sometimes externally blackish – red or covered with "white frost". Seeds 1 ~ 2, reniform, externally brownish – yellow, lustrous, testathin and fragile. Odour of pulp slight; taste sour. Odour of seeds aromatic on crushing; taste pungent and slightly bitter.

2. Microscopic identification

(1)Magnoliae Officinalis Cortex

①Transverse section: Cork consisting of over 10 layers of cells, sometimes rhytidome observed. The outer side of cortex showing a ring of sclereid and the inner side scattered with numerous oil cells and groups of sclereid. Phloem rays 1 ~ 3 cells wide; fibers mostly several in bundles; oil cells scattered.

②Powder: Brown. Fibers numerous, 15 ~ 32μm in diameter, walls strongly thickened, sometimes undulate or serrate at one side, lignified, pit canals indistinct. Sclereidsubsquare, elliptical, ovate, or irregularly branched, 11 ~ 65μm in diameter, sometimes striations visible. Oil cells elliptical or subrounded, 50 ~ 85μm in diameter, containing yellowish – brown oily contents.

(2)Schisandrae Fructus

①Transverse section: Pericarp consisting of 1 layer of square or rectangular epidermal cells, walls relatively thickened, covered with cuticle, oil cells scattered. Mesocarp consisting of 10 or more layers of parenchymatous cells containing starch granules, scattered with small collateral vascular bundles. Endocarp consisting of 1 layer of small square parenchymatous cells. The most outer layer of testa consisting of radially elongated sclereid, thick – walled, with fine and dense pits and pit canals; beneath it showing several layers of sclereid, subrounded, triangular or polygonal with larger pits; underneath the sclereid layers occurring a few layers of parenchymatous cells, vascular bundles occurring in raphes; oil cell layer consisting of 1 layer of rectangular oil cells containing yellowish – brown volatile oil, with 3 ~ 5 layers of small cells lying below; inner epidermal cells of testa small, slightly thick – walled; endosperm cells containing oil droplets and aleurone grains.

②Powder: Sclereid of epidermis of testa polygonal or elongated – polygonal in surface view, 18 ~ 48μm in diameter, walls thickened with very fine and close pit canals, lumen contains dark brown contents. Sclereid of the inner layers of testa polygonal, subrounded or irregular, up to $83\mu m$ in diameter, walls slightly thickened, with relatively large pits. Epidermal cells of pericarp polygonal in surface view, with cuticle striations, scattered with oil cells. Cells of mesocarp shriveled, containing dark brown contents and starch granules.

【Assignments】

1. Make a record and draw the characters of transverse section of Magnoliae Officinalis Cortex.

2. Make a diagram of the characters of powder of Magnoliae Officinalis Cortex.

3. Make a diagram of the transverse section of Schisandrae Chinensis Fructus.

4. Make a diagram of the powder of Schisandrae Chinensis Fructus, and signify the sclereid and the epidermal cells of pericarp.

【Discussion】

1. What parts of the plant does the "bark" crude drugs mainly come from?

2. What the "Nan Wuweizi" (Schisandrae Sphenantherae Fructus) originate from? How to differentiate "Nan Wuweizi" and "Bei Wuweizi" according to their macroscopic characteristics?

实验十六 毛茛科生药——黄连

【实验目的】

1. 掌握黄连的性状、显微鉴别特征。
2. 熟悉根茎类生药的主要鉴别方法。

【实验指导】

毛茛科植物为草本。叶片多缺刻或分裂。花多两性；雄蕊和心皮多数，分离，常螺旋状排列，子房上位。聚合瘦果或聚合蓇葖果。该科来源生药化学成分较复杂，主要含有生物碱、毛茛苷、强心苷等成分。代表生药包括黄连、白芍、赤芍、乌头等。

黄连为毛茛科植物黄连 *Coptis chinensis* Franch.、三角叶黄连 *Coptisdeltoidea* C. Y. Cheng et Hsiao 或云连 *Coptisteeta* Wall. 的干燥根茎。

【仪器与试剂】

1. 仪器
光学显微镜、酒精灯、解剖针、载玻片、盖玻片等。

2. 试剂
水合氯醛溶液、稀甘油、蒸馏水等。

【实验材料】

黄连药材标本及粉末；黄连（根茎）横切面永久制片。

【实验步骤】

1. 性状鉴别
①味连：多集聚成簇，常弯曲，形如鸡爪，单枝根茎长 3~6cm，直径 0.3~0.8cm。表面灰黄色或黄褐色，粗糙，有不规则结节状隆起、须根及须根残基，有的节间表面平滑如茎杆，习称"过桥"。上部多残留褐色鳞叶，顶端常留有残余的茎或叶柄。质坚硬，折断面不整齐，皮部橙红色或暗棕色，木部鲜黄色或橙黄色，呈放射状排列，髓部有时中空。气微，味极苦（图 16-1）。

②雅连：多为单枝，略成圆柱形，微弯曲，长 4~8cm，直径 0.5~1cm。"过桥"较长。顶端有少许残茎。

③云连：弯曲呈钩状，多为单枝，较细小。

2. 显微鉴别
（1）横切面

①味连：木栓层为数列细胞，其外有表皮，常脱落。皮层较宽；石细胞单个或成群散在。中柱鞘纤维成束，或伴有少量石细胞，均显黄色。维管束外韧型，环列。束间形

成层不明显。木质部黄色，均木化，木纤维较发达。髓部由薄壁细胞组成，无石细胞（图16-2）。

②雅连：髓部有石细胞。

③云连：皮层、中柱鞘及髓部均无石细胞。

（2）黄连粉末

石细胞鲜黄色；类圆形、类方形、多角形、类长方形、纺锤形或不规则形；壁厚，有的层纹明显，纹孔细小，孔沟有的分叉；有的石细胞壁较薄，胞腔较大；纤维鲜黄色；韧皮纤维纺锤形或梭形，多成束，有时与石细胞相连结，较粗短，壁厚，胞腔小；木纤维较细长，壁较薄，木化，纹孔稀疏（图16-3）。

【实验报告】

1. 记述三种黄连的性状、组织特征，并绘味连的组织简图。

2. 绘黄连粉末特征图，示石细胞、纤维。

【思考题】

三种商品药材（味连、雅连、云连）在来源、产地上有何不同？

Experiment 16　Identification of Coptidis Rhizoma(Ranunculaceae)

【Objective】

1. To master the macroscopic and microscopic identification of Coptidis Rhizoma.

2. To be familiar with the method of determinaton of crude drugs from plant rhizome.

【Principle】

Ranunculaceae plants are herbaceous. Leaves are often notched or divided. Flowers are mostly bisexual. Stamens and carpels are numerous, separated, and often spirally arranged, ovary superior. Aggregate achenes or follicles. The chemical constituents of this kind of crude drugs are complex, mainly including the alkaloids, buttercup, cardiac glycosides and so on. The representative medicines include Coptidis Rhizoma, Paeoniae Radix Alba, Paeoniae Radix Pubra and Aconiti Radix.

Coptidis Rhizoma is the dried rhizome of *Coptis chinensis* Franch. , *Coptisdeltoidea* C. Y. Cheng et Hsiao or *Coptisteeta* Wall. of Ranunculaceae plants.

【Instruments and Reagents】

1. Instruments

Optical microscope, alcohol lamp, anatomical needle, slide, cover glass.

2. Reagents

Chloral hydrate solution, dilute glycerin, distilled water.

【Materials】

Reference crude drug of Coptidis Rhizoma and its powder; slides of rhizome transverse section of *C. chinensis*, *C. deltoidea* and *C. teeta*.

【Experimental Procedures】

1. Macroscopic identification

（1）Rhizome of *C. chinensis*

Mostly gathered as clusters of curved rhizomes, like "chicken feet", single rhizome 3 ~ 6cm long, 0.3 ~ 0.8cm in diameter. Externally greyish – yellow or yellowish – brown, rough, bearing irregular nodular protrusions, rootlets and remains of rootlets, some internodes smooth as the aerial stem, commonly known as "Guoqiao" (bridge piece). The upper part mostly remains of brown scale leaves, the apex often bearing remains of stems or petioles. Texture hard, fracture uneven, bark orange – red or dark brown, wood brightly yellow or orange – yellow, radially arranged, pith sometimes hollowed. Odour slight; taste very bitter.

（2）Rhizome of *C. deltoidea*

Mostly single, somewhat cylindrical, slightly curved, 4 ~ 8cm long, 0.5 ~ 1cm in diameter. "Guoqiao" relatively long. Apex with some remains of stems.

（3）Rhizome of *C. teeta*

Curved hook – like, mostly single relatively small.

2. Microscopic identification

（1）Transverse section

①Rhizome of *C. chinensis*: Cork cells of several layers. Cortex broader, sclereid singly scattered or grouped. Pericycle Fibers in bundles or accompanied with a few sclereid, both yellow. Collateral vascular bundles arranged in ring. Interfascicular cambium indistinct. Xylem yellow, lignified, xylem fibers well developed. Pith consists of parenchyma cells without sclereid.

②Rhizome of *C. deltoidea*: Pith with sclereid.

③Rhizome of *C. teeta*: Sclereid absent from cortex, pericycle and pith.

（2）Powder

Sclereid bright yellow, subrounded, subsquare, subpolygonal, fusiform or irregular, thick – walled, someone with distinct striations, pits small and pit canals crotched, some with relatively thin walls and large lumina. Fibers bright yellow, phloem fibers long – fusiform or spindle – shaped, mostly in bundles, sometimes connect with sclereid, relatively thick and short, thick – walled, with small lumina. Xylem fibers slender, the walls relatively thin, lignified, pit sparse.

【Assignments】

1. Record the characters of macroscopic and microscopic identification (Transverse section) of the three kinds of Coptidis Rhizoma, and make a diagram of transverse section on Rhizome of *Coptis*

chinensis.

2. Make a diagnostic drawing of power of Coptidis Rhizoma, and signify the sclereid and fibers.

【Discussion】

What're the differences among three commercial drugs(Rhizome of *C. chinensis*, *C. deltoidei* and *C. teeta*)in origin and the producing area?

实验十七　十字花科生药——大青叶

【实验目的】

1. 掌握大青叶的性状及显微鉴别特征。
2. 了解其他大青叶类似生药的植物来源及鉴别特征。

【实验指导】

十字花科植物为草本，植物体有的含辛辣液汁。单叶互生。花两性；花瓣4，十字形排列；雄蕊6，四强；子房上位。本科植物多具乳管或特殊的乳囊组织，含白色乳汁或有色汁液。除少数属外，常不含草酸钙结晶。少数有非腺毛，由1~2列或多列细胞组成；无腺毛，叶表皮的气孔不等式。

大青叶为十字花科植物菘蓝 *Isatisindigotica* Fort. 的干燥叶。

观察叶类生药时，首先将皱缩的叶片湿润展平，再观察叶片的形状、大小、色泽、上下表面、质地以及叶柄的有无或长短等。叶柄若有特征，具有鉴别意义，也需观察和描述。显微鉴定时，通常作横切片观察表皮、叶肉及叶脉的组织构造；或采用表面制片观察表皮细胞、气孔及各种毛茸的形状，以及叶肉组织的某些鉴别点等。应注意上、下表皮细胞的形状，垂周壁，角质层纹理，气孔的型式等。

【仪器与试剂】

1. 仪器
光学显微镜、酒精灯、解剖针、载玻片、盖玻片等。

2. 试剂
水合氯醛溶液、稀甘油、蒸馏水等。

【实验材料】

大青叶药材标本及粉末。

【实验步骤】

1. 性状鉴别
叶多卷曲，暗灰绿色，有时破碎仅剩叶柄。完整叶片呈长椭圆形或宽披针形，长5~20cm，宽2~6cm，先端钝，全缘或微波状，基部狭窄延成翼状叶柄，长4~10cm。质轻易脆。气微，味微酸、苦、涩（图17-1）。

2. 显微鉴别
粉末绿褐色。下表皮细胞垂周壁较为平直或稍弯曲，表面呈连珠状增厚。下表皮气孔较多，不等式；副卫细胞3~4个。叶肉细胞含靛蓝结晶和橙皮苷样结晶。靛蓝结晶蓝色，呈细小颗粒状或片状，长聚集成堆；橙皮苷样结晶淡黄绿色，呈类圆形或不规则形，有的针簇状（图17-2）。

【实验作业】

1. 绘制大青叶叶表皮细胞组织图及气孔图。
2. 以大青叶为例记述叶类生药的鉴别特征。

【思考题】

《中国药典》规定，大青叶为十字花科植物菘蓝 *Isatis indigotica* Fort. 的干燥叶。此外，尚有蓼科植物蓼蓝 *Polygonum tinctorium* Ait. 的干燥叶、爵床科植物马蓝（板蓝）*Strobilanthes cusia*（Nees）Bremek. 的干燥叶、马鞭草科植物路边青（大青）*Clerodendrumcyrtophyllum* Turcz. 的干燥叶，分别为蓼大青叶、马蓝叶和马大青叶，在部分地区当"大青叶"用。如何区别大青叶、蓼大青叶、马蓝叶和马大青叶？

Experiment 17　Identification of Isatidis Folium(Cruciferae)

【Objective】

1. To master the macroscopic and microscopic identification of Isatidis Folium.

2. To understand the origin and identification method of crude drugs which confused with Isatidis Folium.

【Principle】

Cruciferous plants are herbaceous and sometimes contain spicy liquid. Leaves are alternate, flowers bisexual; four pieces of petals, cruciform arranged; tetradynamous stamen, six pieces; ovary superior. Many plants have milk ducts or special milk sacs, containing white milk or colored liquid. Calcium oxalate crystals are usually absent except for a few genera. A few have non – glandular hair, composed of 1 – 2 or more rows of cells; stomatal inequality of leaf epidermis without glandular hairs.

Isatidis Folium is the dried leaf of *Isatis indigotica* Fort. of Cruciferous plants.

To observe the leaf of crude drugs, first the shriveled leaves were wetted and flattened, and then the shape, size, color, upper and lower surfaces, texture and the presence or length of petioles were observed. If the petiole has a characteristic, and the discrimination significance, also needs to observe and the description. In the microscopic identification, the tissue structure of epidermis, mesophyll and vein is usually observed by crosscutting slices. Or observe the shape of epidermal cells, stomata and all kinds of hairy velvet, as well as some identification points of mesophyll tissue. Attention should be paid to the shape of upper and lower epidermal cells, anticlinal wall, cuticle texture, stomatal pattern, etc.

【Instruments and Reagents】

1. Instruments

Optical microscope, alcohol lamp, anatomical needle, slide, cover glass.

2. Reagents

Chloral hydrate solution, dilute glycerin, distilled water.

【Materials】

Reference crude drug of Isatidis Folium and its powder.

【Experimental Procedures】

1. Macroscopic identification

Mostly crumpled and rolled, sometimes broken, dark greyish – green. When intact, long – elliptical to oblong – oblanceolate, 5 ~ 20cm long, 2 ~ 6cm wide; apex obtuse, margin entire or slightly wavy, base attenuated and decurrent to the petiole appearing wing – shaped; petioles 4 ~ 10cm long. Texture fragile. Odour slight; taste slightly sour, bitter and astringent.

2. Microscopic identification

Powder: greenish – brown. Anticlinal walls of epidermal cells rather straight or slightly sinuous, and beaded in surface view. Stomataanomocytic, with 3 ~ 4 subsidiary cells. Mesophyll tissue indistinctly differentiated; mesophyll cells containing blue fine granules and hesperidin – like crystals.

【Assignments】

1. Draw the drafts of leaves epidermal cells and stomata of Isatidis Folium.
2. Record the common characteristic of leaf herb medicine.

【Discussion】

According to the Chinese Pharmacopoeia, the Isatidis Folium is the dried leaf of *Isatis indigotica* Fort. in cruciferous. In addition, the dried leaves of *Polygonum tinctorium* Ait. of Polygonaceae, *Strobilanthescusia* (Nees) Bremek. of Acanthaceae, and *Clerodendrumcyrtophyllum* Turcz. of Verbenaceae also used as "Daqingye" in some areas. How to distinguish Isatidis Folium and the leaves of *Polygonum tinctorium* Ait. , *Baphicacanthuscusia* (Nees) Bremek. , and *Clerodendroncyrtophyllum* Turcz. ?

实验十八　蔷薇科生药——苦杏仁的鉴定

【实验目的】

1. 掌握苦杏仁的性状及显微鉴别特征；
2. 了解与苦杏仁易混淆的其他生药的来源及鉴别方法。

【实验指导】

蔷薇科植物种类多，单叶或复叶，常具托叶。花两性，辐射对称；萼片、花瓣多为 5 基数；蓇葖果、瘦果或梨果。本科生药含有氰苷、多酚、有机酸、黄酮类等成分。代表性生药包括苦杏仁、山楂、郁李仁等。

苦杏仁为蔷薇科植物山杏 *Prunus armeniaca* L. var. *ansu* Maxim.、西伯利亚杏 *Prunus sibirica* L.、东北杏 *Prunus mandshurica*（Maxim.）Koehne 或杏 *Prunus armeniaca* L. 的干燥成熟种子。夏季采收成熟果实，除去果肉和核壳，取出种子，晒干。

种子类生药的鉴别应注意观察其形状、大小、颜色、表面特征、气味等，其中要特别注意其表面特征，如种脐、种脊、合点等特征。种子的构造包括种皮、胚乳和胚。种皮通常包括表皮层、栅状细胞层、油细胞层、色素层、石细胞层等；胚乳分为外胚乳和内胚乳，由薄壁细胞组成，内含大量脂肪油和糊粉粒；胚的大部分通常是子叶，其构造与叶大致相似。显微鉴别时，需重点观察种皮的组织构造、细胞形状等，粉末中种皮表皮碎片的表面观及断面观均可见，注意观察其形态特征。此外，糊粉粒是种仁中贮藏蛋白质的特殊形式，是种子类中药粉末鉴定的主要特征。

【仪器与试剂】

1. 仪器
光学显微镜、酒精灯、解剖针、载玻片、盖玻片等。

2. 试剂
水合氯醛溶液、稀甘油、蒸馏水等。

【实验材料】

苦杏仁药材标本及粉末。

【实验步骤】

1. 性状鉴别
种子呈扁心形，长 1~1.9cm，宽 0.8~1.5cm，厚 0.5~0.8cm。表面黄棕色至红棕色，珠孔位于尖端，近尖端边缘有短线形种脐，钝圆一端较肥厚，有椭圆形合点，种脐与合点间有线形种脊，自合点散出数条深棕色脉纹；种皮与胚乳薄，子叶 2 枚，肥厚，富油性，胚根介于子叶的尖端部分。气微，与水共研可产生苯甲醛香气；味苦（图 18-1）。

83

2. 显微鉴别

粉末黄白色。种皮石细胞单个散在或数个成群，淡黄色或黄棕色。侧面观大多呈贝壳形、类圆形，底部较宽，层纹无或少见，孔沟甚密，上部壁厚 5～10μm，层纹明显，孔沟少；顶面观呈类圆形、类多角形，纹孔大而密（图18-2）。

【实验作业】

绘苦杏仁粉末特征图，示种皮石细胞的顶面观与侧面观。

【思考题】

苦杏仁和桃仁在性状上有何区别？

Experiment 18　Identification of Armeniacae Semen Amarum(Rosaceae)

【**Objective**】

1. To master the macroscopic and microscopic identification of Armeniacae Semen Amarum.

2. To understand the origin and identification method of crude drugs which confused with Armeniacae Semen Amarum.

【**Principle**】

There are many species of Rosaceous plants, simple or compound leaves, often with tubule flowers bisexual, radiation symmetry; sepals petals mostly 5 cardinal; follicles achenes or pear. Raw materials contain cyanosides, polyphenols, organic acids, flavonoids and other components. Representative crude drugs include bitter almond, hawthorn, plum and so on.

Armeniacae Semen Amarum is the dried mature seed of *Prunus armeniaca* L. var. *ansu* Maxim., *Prunus sibirica* L., *Prunus mandshurica* (Maxim.) Koehne and *Prunus armeniaca* L. The ripe fruits are harvested in summer, remove the pulp and shell to get the seeds and then dry them in the sun.

The identification of seeds should pay attention to observe its shape, size, color, surface characteristics, odor and so on, especially for its surface features, such as the hilum, raphe, chalaza, etc. The structure of the seed includes seed coat, endosperm and embryo. Seed coat usually consists of epidermal layer, palisade cell layer, oil cell layer, pigment layer, sclereid layer and other tissues. The endosperm is divided into the outer endosperm and the inner endosperm, and is composed of parenchyma cells containing a large amount of fatty oil and aleurone granules. And the majority of the embryo is usually cotyledon, which are roughly similar in structure to the leaves. For microscopic identification, the histological structure and cell shape of seed coat should be observed, and the surface view and cross section view of the seed coat epidermis fragments were all visible in the micro - characteristics of power. Additionally, aleurone granule is a special form to store protein in seed kernel and is unique in plant organs and is the main feature for seed powder identification.

【Instruments and Reagents】

1. Instruments

Optical microscope, alcohol lamp, anatomical needle, slide, cover glass.

2. Reagents

Chloral hydrate, dilute glycerol, distilled water.

【Materials】

Reference curde drug of Armeniacae Semen Amarum and its powder.

【Experimental Procedures】

1. Macroscopic identification

Flattened – cordate, 1 ~ 1.9cm long, 0.8 ~ 1.5cm wide, 0.5 ~ 0.8cm thick. Externally yellowish brown to deep brown, acute at one end, obtusely rounded plump and unsymmetrical at the other end. A short linear hilum situated at the acute end and a chalaza at the rounded end with numerous upwards deep brown veins. Testa thin; cotyledons 2, milky – white, oily. Odour slight; taste bitter.

2. Microscopic identification

Powder is yellow – white. Sclereid of testa scattered alone or several in groups, pale yellow or yellowish – brown. Almost shell – shaped, subrounded in section view, slightly wide base, without striation or rarely, colporation dense; the upper wall 5 ~ 10μm thick, striation distinct, rare colporation; subrounded, sub – polygonal in surface view, big and dense pit.

【Assignments】

Make a diagnostic drawing of the powdered Armeniacae Semen Amurum, and signify sclereid of testa in surface view and section view.

【Discussion】

How to distinguish Armeniacae Semen Amarum from Persicae Semen via macroscopic characteristics?

实验十九　豆科生药——甘草

【实验目的】

1. 掌握甘草的性状及显微鉴别特征。
2. 了解三种基原甘草的差别。

【实验指导】

豆科植物根部常有根瘤；叶常互生，多为羽状或掌状复叶。具有各种类型的毛茸，腺毛广泛存在。叶表皮气孔常为平轴式。该科来源的生药主要含有黄酮类、生物碱类、三萜类等成分。代表生药包括甘草、黄芪等。

甘草为豆科植物甘草 *Glycyrrhiza uralensis* Fisch. 、胀果甘草 *Glycyrrhiza inflata* Bat. 或光果甘草 *Glycyrrhiza glabra* L. 的干燥根和根茎。

【仪器与试剂】

1. 仪器

光学显微镜、酒精灯、解剖针、载玻片、盖玻片等。

2. 试剂

水合氯醛溶液、稀甘油、蒸馏水等。

【实验材料】

甘草药材标本及粉末，甘草根横切面永久切片。

【实验步骤】

1. 性状鉴别

（1）甘草

根呈圆柱形，长 25～100cm，直径 0.6～3.5cm，外皮松紧不一。表面红棕色或灰棕色，具纵皱纹、皮孔及细根痕。质坚硬，折断面粗纤维性。横切面棕色，形成层环明显，射线放射状。根茎表面有芽痕、疤痕，断面中心有髓。气微，味甜而特殊（图 19-1）。

（2）胀果甘草

根及根茎质地粗壮，有的分枝，外皮粗糙，多灰棕色或灰褐色。质坚硬，木质纤维多，粉性小。根茎不定芽多而粗大。

（3）光果甘草

根及根茎质地较坚实，有的分枝，外皮不粗糙，多灰棕色，皮孔细而不明显。

2. 显微鉴别

（1）根和根茎横切面

木栓层为数列棕色细胞。栓内层较窄。韧皮部射线宽广，多弯曲，常现裂隙；纤维成束，非木化或微木化，周围细胞常含草酸钙方晶；筛管群常因压缩而变形。束内形成层明显。木质部射线宽 3 ~ 5 列细胞；导管较多，直径约至 160μm；木纤维成束，周围细胞含草酸钙方晶。根中心无髓；根茎中心有髓（图 19 - 2）。

（2）粉末

淡棕黄色。纤维成束，直径 8 ~ 14μm，壁厚，微木化，孔沟不明显。晶鞘纤维较多，含晶细胞壁增厚，微木化或非木化。草酸钙方晶呈类双锥形或长方形。具缘纹孔导管较大。木栓细胞呈棕红色，壁薄，微木化，表面观呈多角形（图 19 - 3）。

【实验报告】

1. 绘甘草的根横切面组织简图。
2. 绘甘草粉末特征图，示晶鞘纤维、导管、木栓细胞。

【思考题】

什么是晶鞘纤维？它的特点是什么？

Experiment 19　Identification of Glycyrrhizae Radix et Rhizoma(Leguminosae)

【Objective】

1. To master the macroscopic and microscopic identification of Glycyrrhizae Radix et Rhizoma.

2. To understand the differences among Glycyrrhizae Radix et Rhizoma from *Glycyrrhiza uralensis*, *G. inflata* and *G. glabra*.

【Principle】

Leguminous plants often have root nodules in their roots; leaves often alternate, more pinnate or palmate compound leaves with various types of pilose antlers and widespread glandular hairs. The stomatas of leaf epidermis are usually of the flat axis type. This kind of crude drugs mainly contains the flavonoids, alkaloids, triterpenes and other components. The important drugs from Leguminosae contain Glycyrrhizae Radix et Rhizoma and Astragali Radix, etc.

Glycyrrhizae Radix et Rhizoma is the dried root and rhizome of *Glycyrrhiza uralensis* Fisch. , *Glycyrrhiza inflata* Bat. and *Glycyrrhiza glabra* L. of Leguminous plants.

【Instruments and Reagents】

1. Instruments

Optical microscope, alcohol lamp, anatomical needle, slide, cover glass.

2. Reagents

Chloral hydrate, dilute glycerol, distilled water.

【Materials】

Reference crude drug of Glycyrrhizae Radix et Rhizoma and its powder; slides of root transverse sections of *Glycyrrhizauralensis*.

【Experimental Procedures】

1. Macroscopic identification

（1）Roots of *G. uralensis*

Roots cylindrical, 25 ~ 100cm long, 0. 6 ~ 3. 5cm in diameter. The outer bark loose or tight. Externally reddish – brown or greyish – brown, obviously longitudinally wrinkled, furrowed, lenticel – like protruded, and with sparse rootlet scars. Texture compact, fracture slightly fibrous, yellowish – white, starchy, cambium ring distinct, rays radiate, some with clefts. Rhizomes cylindrical, externally with bud scars, pith present in the center of fracture. Odour, slight; taste, sweet and characteristic.

（2）Roots of *G. inflata*

Roots and rhizomes woody and stout, some branched, the outer bark rough, mostly greyish – brown. Texture compact, lignified fibers abundant, and less starchy. Rhizomes with more and large adventitious buds.

（3）Roots of *G. glabra*

Texture of root and rhizomes relatively compact, some branched, the outer bark not rough, mostly greyish – brown, lenticels small and indistinct.

2. Microscopic identification

（1）Transverse section

Cork consisting of several layers of brown cells. Phelloderm relatively narrow. Phloem rays broad, mostly curved, frequently with clefts; most phloem fibers in bundles, undignified or slightly lignified, surrounded by cells containing prisms of calcium oxalate; sieve tube tissue often pressed to be collapsed. Fascicular cambium distinct. Xylem rays 3 ~ 5 cells wide; vessels frequent, up to $160\mu m$ in diameter; xylem fibers in boundless, surrounded by cells containing prisms of calcium oxalate. Roots without pith at the center; rhizomes possessing pith at the center.

（2）Powder

Pale brownish – yellow. Fibers in bundles, slender, 8 ~ $14\mu m$ in diameter, thick – walled, slightly lignified, surrounded by parenchymatous cells containing prisms of calcium oxalate, forming crystal fibers. Prisms of calcium oxalate frequent. Bordered pitted vessels large. Cork cells reddish – brown, polygonal, slightly lignified.

【Assignments】

1. Make a diagram of the transverse section of Glycyrrhizae Radix et Rhizoma.

2. Make a diagnostic drawing of the powdered Glycyrrhizae Radix et Rhizoma, and signify crystals fibers, cork cells and vessels.

【Discussion】

What is crystalfiber? What are its structural characters?

实验二十 瑞香科生药——沉香

【实验目的】

1. 掌握沉香的性状及显微鉴别特征。
2. 了解不同商品沉香的鉴别特征。

【实验指导】

瑞香科植物多为灌木或乔木。茎皮多韧皮纤维，不易折断。该类生药主要含有二萜酯类、香豆素类、木脂素类、挥发油和黄酮类等成分。代表生药包括沉香、芫花等。

沉香为瑞香科植物白木香 *Aquilaria sinensis*（Lour.）Gilg 含有树脂的木材。

进口沉香为瑞香科植物沉香 *Aquilariaagallocha* Roxb. 含有树脂的心材。

【仪器与试剂】

1. 仪器
光学显微镜、酒精灯、解剖针、载玻片、盖玻片等。

2. 试剂
水合氯醛溶液、稀甘油、蒸馏水等。

【实验材料】

沉香药材标本及粉末；沉香三切面永久切片。

【实验步骤】

1. 性状鉴别

（1）沉香（白木香）

呈不规则块状、片状或盔帽状，有的为小碎块；表面凹凸不平，有刀痕，偶有孔洞，可见黑褐色树脂与黄白色木部相间的斑纹，孔洞及凹窝表面多呈朽木状。质较坚实，断面刺状。气芳香，味苦（图 20 - 1）。

（2）进口沉香

呈圆柱形或不规则块片，两端或表面有刀劈痕、沟槽或孔洞，凹凸不平；表面淡黄色或灰黑色，密布断续的棕黑色纵纹（含树脂的木射线），有时可见黑褐色树脂斑痕，微具光泽，横断面可见细密棕黑色斑点。质坚硬而重，能沉或半沉于水。气味较浓烈（图 20 - 2）。

2. 显微鉴别

（1）国产沉香切面

①横切面：木射线宽 1 ~ 2 列细胞，含棕色树脂；导管圆多角形，直径 42 ~ 128μm，有的含棕色树脂；木纤维多角形，直径 20 ~ 45μm，壁稍厚，木化；木间韧皮部扁长椭圆形或条带状，常与射线相交，细胞壁薄，内含棕色树脂；其间散有少数纤维（图 20 - 3A）。

②径向纵切面：射线呈条带状，细胞同型（图 20 - 3B）。

③切向纵切面：射线高 4 ~ 15 个细胞；导管具缘纹孔排列紧密；木间韧皮部细胞类长方形（图 20 – 3C）。

（2）国产沉香粉末

纤维管胞多成束，长梭形，壁较薄，径向壁上有具缘纹孔。导管具缘纹孔排列紧密，内含黄棕色树脂块。木射线细胞壁连珠状增厚。树脂团块黄棕色（图 20 – 4）。

【实验报告】

描述国产沉香三个切面组织特征。

【思考题】

1. 鉴定木类药材三切面时，各切面分别可以观察哪些特征？
2. 进口沉香与国产沉香有何不同？

Experiment 20 Identification of Aquilariae Lignum Resinatum(Thymelaeaceae)

【Objective】

1. To master the macroscopic and microscopic identification of Aquilariae Lignum Resinatum.
2. To study the characters of different commercial Aquilariae Lignum Resinatum.

【Principle】

Thymelaeaceae are mostly shrubs or trees. Stem bark bast fiber, not easy to break. The crude drugs mainly contain diterpenes, coumarins, lignans, essential oils and flavonoids. On behalf of the raw medicine including white wood incense, flowers, such as Genkwa.

Aquilariae Lignum Resinatum is the resin – contained wood of *Aquilaria sinensis* (Lour.) Gilg, Imported Aquilariae is the resin – contained wood of *Aquilaria agallocha* Roxb. Both of them are from Thymelaeaceae.

【Instruments and Reagents】

1. Instruments
Optical microscope, alcohol lamp, anatomical needle, slide, cover glass.

2. Reagents
Chloral hydrate, dilute glycerol, distilled water.

【Materials】

Reference curde drug of Aquilariae Lignum Resinatum and its powder. Slides of stem tansverse section, radial longitudinal section and tangential longitudinal section of heartwood of *Aquilaria sinensis*.

【Experimental Procedures】

1. Macroscopic identification

（1）Chinese eaglewood wood

In irregular lumps and flakes, or helmet – shaped, sometimes in shreds. Externally lumpy, with scars of knife cutting, and showing a few of holes, and streaks formed by black – brown resin alternating with yellowish – white wood. Surface of holes and depressions mostly rotten wood – like. Texture relatively compact, fracture splintery. Odour aromatic; taste bitter. Rotten wood.

（2）Foreign eaglewood wood

In irregular lumps and flakes or cylindrical. Externally and amphi – lumpy, with scars of knife cutting, furrow, and a few holes, externally black – brown or gray – black, densely covered brown – black longitudinal striation interruptedly, and scars of black – brown resin, with burnish slightly, meticulous brown – black spot in transection. Texture relatively pachy and heavy, sagging or floating in water. Odour relatively intensity.

2. Microscopic identification

（1）Section of Chinese eaglewood wood

①Transverse section：Xylem rays 1 ~ 2 cells wide, filled with brown resin. Vessels round – polygonal, 42 ~ 128 μm in diameter, someone's containing brown resin. Xylem fibers polygonal, 20 ~ 45 μm in diameter, with slightly thickened and lignified walls. Interxylary phloem elongated – elliptical or strip – shaped, usually intersecting with rays, and the cells with thin walls, containing brown resin, a few of fibers scattered.

②Vertical longitudinal section：Ray long about 4 ~ 15 cells, vessels pits arranged tightly; liber cells rectangle similarity.

③Radial longitudinal section：Ray strip – shaped, cells homeotype.

（2）Powder

Fibers tracheid fasciculation mostly, fusiform shape, wall usually thinner, with pit in radial wall. Vessels' pits arranged tightly, and yellowish – brown resin lump. Xylem ray cells wall beaded thickening. Resin mass yellowish – brown.

【Assignments】

Record the characters of three issue sections of *Aquilaria sinensis*（Lour.）Gilg.

【Discussion】

1. What characters can be seen in the three different sections of lignum?

2. What are the differences between foreign eaglewood wood and Chinese eaglewood wood?

实验二十一　五加科生药——人参、三七

【实验目的】

1. 掌握人参、三七的性状及显微鉴别特征。
2. 了解常见的人参伪品与人参在性状和显微特征方面的主要鉴别点。

【实验指导】

五加科植物多为木本，稀多年生草本。叶多互生。花两性。浆果或核果。本科植物常有长而硬的单列或成二歧、丛生、星状与盾状的非腺毛。气孔常为平轴式。分泌道常见，多存在于皮层、韧皮部和髓部，某些属植物的射线中有胞间性分泌道。草酸钙簇晶较常见，亦有方晶。本科生药化学成分主要有皂苷类、黄酮及其苷类、香豆素类等。代表性生药有人参、三七、五加皮、竹节参等。

人参为五加科植物人参 *Panax ginseng* C. A. Mey. 的干燥根和根茎。

三七为五加科植物三七 *Panax notoginseng*（Burk.）F. H. Chen 的干燥根和根茎。

【仪器与试剂】

1. 仪器
光学显微镜、解剖针、载玻片、盖玻片等。

2. 试剂
水合氯醛溶液、稀甘油、蒸馏水等。

【实验材料】

人参、三七的药材标本及粉末；人参根横切片永久制片。

【实验步骤】

1. 性状鉴别

（1）人参

①生晒参：主根圆柱形或纺锤形，表面黄白色或淡黄白色，上部有断续粗横纹，全体具明显的纵皱纹，须根上有不明显的疣状突起（习称"珍珠疙瘩"）。根茎（习称"芦头"）较短细，具茎痕（习称"芦碗"）及不定根（习称"艼"）。主根质硬，断面淡黄白色，形成层环棕黄色，皮部有黄棕色点状树脂道及放射状裂隙。香气特异；味微苦、甘（图 21-1）。

②红参：主根圆柱形或纺锤形，表面棕红色，半透明，有时上部棕黄色；有纵沟、皱纹及细根痕；质硬脆，断面平坦，角质样，中心色较浅。

③生晒山参：主根与根茎等长或稍短，表面灰黄色，有浅皱纹，上部有细密环纹。根茎具多数密集的芦碗和艼，须根具较多而明显的珍珠疙瘩。常以"芦长碗密枣核艼，紧皮

细纹珍珠须"概括其性状特征。

（2）三七

①主根：呈类圆锥形或圆柱形，长 1～6cm，直径 1～4cm。表面灰褐色或灰黄色，有断续的纵皱纹和支根痕。顶端有茎痕，周围有瘤状突起。体重，质坚实，断面灰绿色、黄绿色或灰白色，木部微呈放射状排列。气微，味苦回甜（图 21－2）。

②筋条：呈圆柱形或圆锥形，长 2～6cm，上端直径约 0.8cm，下端直径约 0.3cm。

③剪口：呈不规则的皱缩块状或条状，表面有数个明显的茎痕及环纹，断面中心灰绿色或白色，边缘深绿色或灰色。

2. 显微鉴别

（1）人参

①横切面：生晒参主根横切面（图 21－3）：木栓层为数列细胞。栓内层窄。韧皮部外侧有裂隙，内侧薄壁细胞排列较紧密，有树脂道散在（图 21－4），内含黄色分泌物。形成层成环。木质部射线宽广，导管单个散在或数个相聚，断续排列成放射状，导管旁偶有非木化的纤维。薄壁细胞含草酸钙簇晶（图 21－5）。

②粉末：树脂道碎片易见，内含黄色块状分泌物。草酸钙簇晶直径 20～86μm，多数棱角锐尖。木栓细胞表面观呈类方形或多角形，垂周壁细波状弯曲。导管主为网纹及梯纹导管（图 21－6）。

（2）三七

本品粉末灰黄色。淀粉粒甚多，单粒圆形、半圆形或圆多角形，直径 4～30μm；复粒由 2～10 余分粒组成。树脂道碎片含黄色分泌物。梯纹导管、网纹导管及螺纹导管直径 15～55μm。草酸钙簇晶少见，直径 50～80μm（图 21－7）。

3. 常见人参伪品的鉴别

（1）商陆

为商陆科植物商陆 *Phytolacca acinosa* Roxb. 或垂序商陆 *P. americana* L. 的根。表面红棕色或棕褐色。无芦头而有茎的残基。商陆根横切面木栓层多已除去，有同心性排列的三生维管束。有的薄壁细胞含草酸钙针晶。无草酸钙簇晶及树脂道。

（2）华山参

为茄科植物漏斗泡囊草 *Physochlainainfundibularis* Kuang 的根。有短根茎，但无芦碗。表面黄棕色，具点状须根痕。华山参根横切面，残存的木栓层含棕色物。次生皮层及韧皮薄壁细胞含草酸钙砂晶。无树脂道与草酸钙簇晶，具生物碱反应，有毒。

（3）野豇豆

为豆科植物野豇豆 *Vigna vexillata*（Linn.）Rich. 的根。野豇豆根表面灰棕色，有显著纵纹，无横纹，有豆腥气。木栓层多已除去。皮部、木部均含有纤维，不含草酸钙簇晶。

（4）土人参

为马齿苋科植物锥花土人参 *Talinum paniculatum*（Jacq.）Gaertn. 的根。土人参根端有残茎而无芦头、芦碗，质坚实，断面平坦，中央常有大空腔，有的薄壁细胞含草酸钙簇晶，但无树脂道。

【实验报告】

1. 绘人参、三七根横切面组织简图。

2. 绘人参粉末的草酸钙簇晶、树脂道碎片图。

3. 绘三七粉末显微特征图。

【思考题】

人参的草酸钙簇晶与大黄的草酸钙簇晶有什么区别?

Experiment 21 Identification of Ginseng Radix et Rhizoma and Notoginseng Radix et Rhizoma(Araliaceae)

【Objective】

1. To master the macroscopic and microscopic identification of Ginseng Radix et Rhizoma and Notoginseng Radix et Rhizoma.

2. To understand the distinguishing characters of *P. ginseng* and its adulterants.

【Principle】

Araliaceae plants are mostly woody, rare perennial herbs. Leaves are alternate. Flowers bisexual. Berries or drupes. Plants often have long hard single rows or bifid, fascicled, stellate, or shield non – glandular hairs. Stomata are usually of the flat axis type. The secretory tract is common, mainly exists in the cortex, phloem and pith, and there is intercellular secretory tract in the rays of some genera. Calcium oxalate cluster crystals are more common, there are also square crystals. The main phytochemical components are saponins, flavones and their glycosides, coumarins, etc. The representative crude drugs are Ginseng Radix et Rhizoma, Notoginseng Radix et Rhizoma, Acanthopanacis Cortex, Panacis Japonici Rhizoma and so on.

Ginseng Radix et Rhizoma is the dried root and rhizome of *Panax ginseng* C. A. Mey. of Araliaceae plants. Notoginseng Radix et Rhizoma is the dried root and rhizome of *Panax notoginseng* (Burk.)F. H. Chen of Pentacaceae plants.

【Instruments and Reagents】

1. Instruments
Optical microscope, alcohol lamp, anatomical needle, slide, cover glass.

2. Reagents
Chloral hydrate, dilute glycerol, distilled water.

【Materials】

Reference crude drugs of Ginseng Radix et Rhizoma and Notoginseng Radix et Rhizoma and their powders; sildes of root transverse section of *Panax ginseng*.

【Experimental Procedures】

1. Macroscopic identification

（1）Ginseng Radix et Rhizoma

①White Ginseng：Main roots fusiform or cylindrical，externally greyish – yellow；upper part or entire root exhibiting sparse，shallow，interrupted rootlets and coarse transverse – striations and distinct longitudinal wrinkles；numerous slender rootlets with inconspicuous minute tubercles（Zhenzhugeda）. Rhizomes（Lutou）mostly constricted and curved，bearing adventitious roots（Ding）and sparse depressed circular stem scars（Luwan）. Texture relatively hard，fracture yellowish – white，cambium ring brownish – yellow，bark exhibiting yellow – brown dotted resin canals and radial clefts. Odour slight；taste slightly bitter and sweet.

②Red Ginseng：Main roots fusiform or cylindrical. Externally reddish – brown with translucent，occasionally exhibiting a few yellowish – brown；furrowed，longitudinal wrinkles and rootlet scars，the upper part exhibiting interrupted indistinct annulations. Texture hard and fragile，fracture even，horny.

③Dried Wild Ginseng：Main roots as long as or shorter than rhizome，externally greyish – yellow，longitudinally wrinkled，upper end with dense deep depressed annulations. Rhizome with numerous dense stem scars（Luwan）and adventitious roots（Ding），rootlets orderly arranged and showing some distinct warts，known as "pearl – like knot"（Zhenzhugeda）.

（2）Notoginseng Radix et Rhizoma

①Main roots：Subconical or cylindrical，1~6cm long，1~4cm in diameter. Externally greyish – brown or greyish – yellow with interrupted longitudianl wrinkles and branch root scars. Stem scars at the apex surrounded by warty protrudings. Texture heavy and campact，fracture greyish – green，yellowish – green or greyish – white，wood slightly radially arranged. Odour slight；taste bitter but afterwards sweetish.

②Jintiao：Cylindrical or conical，2~6cm long，the upper end 0.8cm in diameter，the lowerend 0.3cm in diameter.

③Jiankou：Irregularly shrunken lump – shaped or slat – shaped，externally with several conspicuous stem scars and annulations；fracture greyish – green or greyish – white in the centre and deep green or grey at the margin.

2. Microscopic identification

（1）Ginseng Radix et Rhizoma

①Transverse section：Cork consisting of several rows of cells. Phelloderm narrow. Phloem showing clefts in the outer part，parenchymatous cells densely arranged and scattered with resin canals containing yellow secretions in the inner part. Cambium in a ring. Xylem rays broad，vessels singly scattered or grouped，interruptedly arranged radially，occasionally accompanied by non – lignified fibres. Parenchymatous cells containing clusters of calcium oxalate.

②Powder：Fragments of resin canals containing yellow masses of secretion. Clusters of calcium oxalate 20~86μm in diameter，with acute angles. Cork cells subsquare or polygonal，with thin and sinuous walls. Reticulate and scalariform vessels.

（2）Notoginseng Radix et Rhizoma

Powder：Greyish – yellow. Starch granules fairly abundant, simple granules rounded, semispherical or round – polygonal, 4 ~ 30μm in diameter；compound granules consisting of 2 ~ 10 or more components. Fragments of resin canals containing yellow secretion. Scalariform, reticulated and spiral vessels 15 ~ 55μm in diameter. Clusters of calcium oxalate infrequent, 50 ~ 80μm in diameter.

3. Identification of the adulterants of Ginseng Radix et Rhizoma

（1）Phytolaccae Radix

The dried root of *Phytolacca acinosa* Roxb or *P. americana* L. Externally reddish brown or dark brown. Without rhizomes（Lutou）but bearing remains of stems. Transverse section of root, most cork removed. Fibro – vascular tissue forming tertiary structure, with several concentric cambium rings. Parenchymatous cells containing raphides of calcium oxalate, not containing clusters of calcium oxalate and resin canals.

（2）Physochlainae Radix

The dried root of *Physochlainainfundibularis* Kuang, family Solanaceae. Bearing short rhizoma without stem stars（Luwan）, Externally yellowish brown, some rootlet scars appearing on the upper part. Transverse section of root with remains of cork containing brown substances. Secondary cortex and phloem parenchymatous cells containing sandy crystals of calcium oxalate, not containing clusters of calcium oxalate and resin canals. Alkaloid reaction is positive. Poisonous.

（3）Vignae Vexillatae Radix

The dried root of *Vigna vexillata*（Linn.）Rich, family Leguminosae. Externally grayish brown with distinct longitudinal wrinkles without transversal wrinkles. Odour, bean – like. Most cork removed. Both bark and wood containing fibers, not containing clusters of calcium oxalate.

（4）Talini Paniculati Radix

The dried root of *Talinum paniculatum*（Jacq.）Gaertn, family Portulacaceae. The upper part bearing the remains of stem, without rhizomes（Lutou）, depressed circular stem scars（Luwan）, texture hard, fracture fairly even, the center usually hollowed. Parenchymatous cells sometimes containing clusters of calcium oxalate, not containing resin canals.

【Assignments】

1. Make a diagram of the transverse section of Ginseng Radix et Rhizoma and Notoginseng Radix et Rhizoma.

2. Make a drawing of the powder of Ginseng Radix et Rhizoma, and signify clusters of calcium oxalate and resin canals.

3. Make a drawing of the powder of Notoginseng Radix et Rhizoma.

【Discussion】

What are the differences between the clusters of calcium oxalate in Ginseng Radix et Rhizoma and Rhei Radix et Rhizoma?

实验二十二　伞形科生药——当归、小茴香

【实验目的】

1. 掌握当归和小茴香的性状及显微鉴别特征。
2. 熟悉当归和小茴香的化学成分。

【实验指导】

伞形科植物为草本，常含挥发油而有香气。茎中空，表面常有纵棱。叶互生，复叶或羽状分裂；叶柄基部扩大成鞘状；花小，两性或杂性，多辐射对称；花瓣5；雄蕊5，与花瓣互生；子房下位。双悬果，外果皮表面有棱和沟槽。本科植物常有分泌道。

当归为伞形科植物当归 *Angelica sinensis*（Oliv.）Diels 的干燥根。小茴香为伞形科植物茴香 *Foeniculum vulgare* Mill. 的干燥成熟果实。

【仪器与试剂】

1. 仪器
光学显微镜、酒精灯、解剖针、载玻片、盖玻片。

2. 试剂
水合氯醛溶液、稀甘油、蒸馏水等。

【实验材料】

当归、小茴香药材标本及粉末；当归根横切面永久制片；小茴香果实横切面永久制片。

【实验步骤】

1. 性状鉴别

（1）当归

根头（归头）及主根（归身）粗短，略成圆柱形，支根（归尾）3～5条或更多，扭曲。表面浅棕色至棕褐色，有纵皱纹及横向皮孔，根头上端圆钝，残留多层鳞片状叶鞘残基。支根上粗下细，多扭曲，有少数须根痕。质较柔软，断面黄白色或淡黄棕色，皮部有多数棕色油点，形成层环黄棕色。有浓郁的香气，味甘、辛、微苦（图22－1）。

（2）小茴香

本品为双悬果，呈圆柱形，有的稍弯曲，长4～8mm，直径1.5～2.5mm。表面黄绿色或淡黄色，两端略尖，顶端残留黄棕色突起的柱基，基部有时有细果柄。悬果瓣（分果）呈长椭圆形，背面有纵棱5条，接合面平坦；横切面略呈五边形，背面的四边约等长。香气特异，味微甜、辛（图22－2）。

2. 显微鉴别

（1）当归

①横切面：当归根横切面（图22－3）：木栓层为数列木栓细胞。皮层窄，有少数油

室。韧皮部宽广，多裂隙，油室（图22 –4）或油管类圆形，直径25～160μm，外侧较大，向内渐小，周围分泌细胞6～9个。形成层成环。木质部射线宽3～5列细胞；导管单个散在或2～3个相聚，呈放射状排列；薄壁细胞含淀粉粒。

②粉末：淡黄棕色。韧皮薄壁细胞纺锤形，壁稍厚，表面有微细斜向交错的纹理，有时可见菲薄的横隔。梯纹及网纹导管多见，直径约至80μm。油室碎片有时可见（图22 –5）。

（2）小茴香

分果横切面：外果皮为1列扁平细胞，外被角质层。中果皮纵棱处有维管束，其周围有多数木化网纹细胞；背面纵棱间各有大的椭圆形棕色油管1个，接合面有油管2个，共6个（图22 –6）。内果皮为1列扁平薄壁细胞，细胞长短不一。种皮细胞扁长，含棕色物。胚乳细胞多角形，含多数糊粉粒，每个糊粉粒中含有细小草酸钙簇晶（图22 –7）。

【实验报告】

1. 记述当归和小茴香的组织特征，绘制当归横切面、小茴香分果的横切面组织简图。
2. 记述当归粉末特征，绘韧皮薄壁细胞图。

【思考题】

1. 归头、归身、归尾各属当归哪个部位？各在功效上有何区别？以何地产者为道地药材？
2. 什么是镶嵌细胞？

Experiment 22　Identification of Angelicae Sinensis Radix and Foeniculif Fructus(Umbelliferae)

【Objective】

1. To master the macroscopic and microscopic identification of Angelicae Sinensis Radix and Foeniculi Fructus.

2. To master the chemical constituents of Angelicae Sinensis Radix and Foeniculi Fructus.

【Principle】

Plants of Umbelliferae family are herbaceous and often contain volatile oil. Stem hollow and the surface often has longitudinal edge. Leaves are alternate, leaf blade compound or pinnately divided; petiole usually sheathing at base; flowers are small, bisexual or heterozygous, and radiosymmetric. Petals 5; stamens 5, alternate with petals; inferior ovary. Double suspended fruit, with ribs and grooves on surface. Plants of Umbelliferae usually have secretory pathways.

Angelicae Sinensis Radix is the dried root of *Angelicae sinensis*(Oliv.)Diels in Umbelliferae. Foeniculi Fructus is the dried ripe fruit of *Foeniculum vulgare* Mill. in Umbelliferae.

【Instruments and Reagents】

1. Instruments

Optical microscope, alcohol lamp, anatomical needle, slide, cover glass.

2. Reagents

Chloral hydrate, dilute glycerol, distilled water.

【Materials】

Reference crude drugs of Angelicae sinensis Radix and Foeniculi Fructus, and their powders; slides of root of *Angelicae sinensis*; slides of fruit of *Foeniculum vulgare*.

【Experimental Procedures】

1. Macroscopic identification

(1) Angelicae Sinensis Radix

Somewhat cylindrical, the root stock known as "Guitou", main root known as "Guishen", the branching root 3 ~ 5, twist, called "Guiwei". Externally yellowish – brown to dark brown, longitudinally wrinkled and transversely lenticellate; the upper portion swollen, blunt and rounded, showing remains of stem and leaf sheaths; branching root, thick in the upper portion and thin in the lower portion, mostly twisted and exhibiting a few rootlet scars. Texture flexible, fracture yellowish – white or yellowish – brown, bark thick, showing brown oil spots, cambium ring yellowish – brown. Odour, strongly aromatic; taste, sweet, pungent and slightly bitter.

(2) Foeniculi Fructus

Cremocarp, elliptical, some slightly curved, 4 ~ 8mm long, 1.5 ~ 2.5mm in diameter. Externally yellowish – green or pale yellow, tapering slightly towards both ends, apex bearing remains of yellowish – brown projecting stylopodium, having a small fruit stalk at the base. Mericarp elongated – elliptical, with each dorsal surface bearing five ribs and commissural surface flattened and broad. Transverse section showing a pentagonal, the four sides of dorsal surface nearly equal in length. Odour, characteristically aromatic; taste, slightly sweet and pungent.

2. Microscopic identification

(1) Angelicae Sinensis Radix

①Transverse section: Cork cells in several layers. Cortex narrow, scattered with a few oil cavities. Phloem broad, more cleft, oil cavities or oil tubes subrounded, 25 ~ 160μm in diameter, relatively large on the outer side, gradually becoming small inwards, surrounded by 6 ~ 9 secretory cells. Cambium in a ring. Xylem rays 3 ~ 5 rows of cells wide; vessels arranged radiatively.

②Powder: Pale yellowish – brown, parenchymatous cells in phloem fusiform, walls slightly thickened, with very fine oblique crisscross striations, sometimes thin transverse septa visible. Scalariform and reticulate vessels frequent, up to 80μm in diameter. Sometimes fragments of oil cavities visible.

(2) Foeniculi Fructus

Transverse section: Exocarp consisting of 1 layer of flattened cells, covered with cuticle at outside. Mesocarp with 5 ribs, each containing a vascular bundle surrounded by numerous lignified reticulate cells. Vittae 6, large, elliptical and brown, 4 of them situated in the dorsal between every 2 ribs and 2 in the commissural. Endocarp consisting of 1 layer of flattened thin – walled cells varying in length. The testa cells compressed and elongated, containing brown contents. Endosperm cells polygonal, filled with aleurone grains, each embedding a minute cluster of calcium oxalate.

【Assignments】

1. Record the characters of transverse section of Angelicae Sinensis Radix and Foeniculi Fructus, and draw their diagram.

2. Record the characters of powder of Angelicae Sinensis Radix, and make a drawing of parenchymatous cells in phloem.

【Discussion】

1. Which parts do "Guitou", "Guishen" and "Guiwei" belong to respectively? What are the differences among the three on effect? Where is the genuine crude drug from?

2. What is incrusted cell?

实验二十三　唇形科生药——薄荷、丹参

【实验目的】

1. 掌握薄荷、丹参的性状及显微鉴别特征。
2. 了解唇形科生药的主要鉴别特征。

【实验指导】

唇形科植物为草本，常含挥发油，气芳香。茎四棱形。多单叶对生。轮伞花序，有的再组成复合花序；花两性，两侧对称，花萼 5 裂，二唇形，宿存；花冠多为二唇形；二强雄蕊；子房上位；果为 4 枚小坚果。本科植物具厚角组织、直轴式气孔；具有腺毛、腺鳞和非腺毛。本科生药含挥发油、二萜（醌）类、黄酮类等成分。代表性生药有薄荷、丹参、黄芩等。

薄荷为唇形科植物薄荷 *Mentha haplocalyx* Briq. 的干燥地上部分。丹参为唇形科植物丹参 *Salvia miltiorrhiza* Bge. 的干燥根和根茎。

【仪器与试剂】

1. 仪器

光学显微镜、酒精灯、解剖针、载玻片、盖玻片等。

2. 试剂

水合氯醛溶液、稀甘油、蒸馏水等。

【实验材料】

薄荷药材标本及其茎、叶横切面永久制片；丹参药材标本及其粉末；丹参根永久切片。

【实验步骤】

1. 性状鉴别

（1）薄荷

茎呈方柱形，有时对生分枝；表面紫棕色或淡绿色，有明显的节，节间长 2 ~ 5cm；棱角处有柔毛；质脆，断面白色，中空。叶卷曲皱缩，长椭圆形或卵形，有凹点状腺鳞。茎上部腋生轮伞花序，花冠多数存在，淡紫色。叶揉搓时有特异清凉的香气；味辛凉。

（2）丹参

根呈长圆柱形，有的分支具须状细根，长 10 ~ 20cm；表面棕红色或暗棕红色，具纵皱纹；老根表面紫棕色，常成鳞片状脱落；质脆，断面疏松，皮部棕红色；气微，味微苦涩（图 23 - 1）。

2. 显微鉴别

（1）薄荷

①茎横切面：呈四方形，表皮为 1 列长方形细胞；皮层薄壁细胞数列，排列疏松，四

棱角处由厚角细胞组成；内皮层明显，韧皮部狭窄，形成层成环。木质部在四棱处发达。髓薄壁细胞大，中心常有空洞（图23-2）。

②叶横切面：上表皮细胞呈长方形，下表皮细胞细小扁平，有气孔；上下表皮有多数凹陷，内有大型特异的扁球形腺鳞。叶肉栅栏组织1~2列细胞，海绵组织为4~5列细胞，叶肉细胞含针簇状橙皮苷结晶。主脉维管束外韧型，韧皮部和木质部外侧有厚角组织（图23-3）。

③叶表面观：腺鳞头部8细胞，直径约至90μm，柄单细胞；小腺毛头部及柄部均为单细胞；非腺毛1~8细胞，常弯曲，壁厚，微具疣突；下表皮气孔多见，直轴式。

（2）丹参

①根横切面：韧皮部较宽广，呈半月形；形成层成环，束间形成层不甚明显；木质部数束，呈放射状；导管在形成层处较多，渐至中央导管呈单列。木部纤维成束存在于中央的初生木质部（图23-4）。

②粉末：红棕色。石细胞类圆形、类三角形、类长方形或不规则形，也有延长呈纤维状，边缘不平整，直径14~70μm，长可达257μm，孔沟明显，有的胞腔内含黄棕色物。木纤维多为纤维管胞，长梭形，末端斜尖或钝圆，直径12~27μm，具缘纹孔点状，纹孔斜裂缝状或十字形，孔沟稀疏。网纹导管和具缘纹孔导管直径11~60μm（图23-5）。

【实验报告】

1. 绘薄荷茎横切面简图及叶表面显微特征图，示腺鳞、非腺毛、表皮细胞及气孔。
2. 记录丹参显微特征图。

【思考题】

1. 唇形科全草类生药有哪些共同的性状与显微特征？
2. 双子叶植物草质茎的次生构造与木质茎的主要区别是什么？

Experiment 23　Identification of Menthae Haplocalycis Herba and Salviae Miltiorrhizae Radix et Rhizoma(Lamiaceae)

【Objective】

1. To master the macroscopic and microscopic identification of Menthae Haplocalycis Herba and Salviae Miltiorrhizae Radix et Rhizoma.

2. To be familiar with the main characteristics of crude drugs from Family Labiatae.

【Principle】

The Labiatae Family is herbaceous, containing volatile oil, aromatic. Stems are quadrangular. Simple leaves, inflorescences areverticillaes, some reconstituting terminal or axillary racemes, capitulum, spica, or panicle; flowers are bisexual, bilaterally symmetric, calyx five - parted and bilabiate; bilabiate corollas; didynamous, the ovary is superior. The fruits are four small nuts. The plants of this family have collenchyma and straight – axis stomata; and has glandular hairs, glandular scales and non – glandular hairs. And contain volatile oil, diterpenes (quinones), flavonoids and other components. Representative crude drugs include Menthae Haplocalycis Herba, Salviae Miltiorrhizae Radix et Rhizoma and so on.

Menthae Haplocalycis Herba is the dried overground part of *Mentha haplocalyx*biq. (Family Lamiaceae). Salviae Miltiorrhizae Radix et Rhizoma is the dried root and rhizome of *Salvia miltiorrhiza* Bunge(Family Lamiaceae).

【Instruments and Reagents】

1. Instruments

Optical microscope, alcohol lamp, anatomical needle, slide, cover glass.

2. Reagents

Chloral hydrate, dilute glycerol, distilled water.

【Materials】

Reference crude drugs of Menthae Haplpcalycis Herba and Salviae Miltiorrhizae Radix et Rhizoma, and their powders. Sildes of stem and leaf transverse section of *Mentha haplocalyx*; sildes of root transverse section of *Salvia miltiorrhiza*.

【Experimental Procedures】

1. Macroscopic identification

(1)Menthae Haplpcalycis Herba

Stem square, sometimes with opposite branches; externally purplish – brown or light green, with distinct nodes, internodes 2 ~ 5cm long; the angular regions pubescent; texture fragile, fracture white, pith hollowed. Lamina crumpled and rolled, long – elliptical or ovate, bearing concave dotted grandular scales. Verticillaster axillary, coralla mostly existing, pale purple. Odour, characteristic and aromatic after rubbing leaves; taste, pungent and cool.

(2)Salviae Miltiorrhizae Radix et Rhizoma

Roots long cylindrical, some branches with fibrous roots are 10 ~ 20cm long; surface brownish – red or dark brown – red, with longitudinal wrinkles; old roots surface is purplish – brown, often scale – like exfoliation; bark brownish – red; taste slightly bitter and astringent.

2. Microscopic identification

(1)Menthae Haplpcalycis Herba

①Transverse section of stem: Square. Epidermal cells, rectangle, 1 layer. Parenchymatous cells, several layers, arranged laxly, four angular regions consisting of collenchyma cells. Endodermis pubescent. Phloem narrow. Cambium in ring. Xylem developed on the four angular regions. Parenchymatous cells of pith large, pith often hollowed.

②Transverse section of leaf: The upper epidermal cells, rectangle, the lower epidermal cells small and flattened, with stomata; the upper and lower epidermis numerously pitted, with large and characteristic flattened – spherical glandular scales. Palisade tissue consisting of 1 ~ 2 layers' cells, spongy tissue 4 ~ 5 layers of cells, mesophyll tissue containing needle – clusters of hesperidin. Vascular bundles of main vein collateral, collenchyma tissue on the out – side of phloem and xylem.

③Surface view of leaf:8 cells in the head of glandular scale, up to 90μm in diameter, single cell in stalk. The head and stalk of small glandular hair are all single cells. Non – glandular hairs 1 ~ 8 cells, often curved, walls thick, small vertussis; stomata of lower epidermis are more common, straight axis type.

(2)Salviae Miltiorrhizae Radixet Rhizoma

①Transverse section of root:Phloem is broad and half – moon shaped; the cambium was ringed and the interfascicular cambium was not obvious. Xylem several beams, radiating; conduits in cambium, and the central catheter is a single row gradually. Fascicles of wood fibers exist in the central primary xylem.

②Powder:Reddish – brown, sclereids are round, subtriangular, oblong, or irregular in shape, or elongate to be fibrous, with uneven edges, 14 ~ 17μm in diameter, up to 257μm in length, obvious pores and grooves, and some cells contain yellowish – brown materials. Most of the wood fibers are fibrous cells, long spindle shaped, with obtuse or obtuse ends, 12 ~ 27μm in diameter, with pointy marginal orifice, oblique fissure, or cross shaped orifice, with sparse orifice. Reticulated and margined orifice conduits are 11 ~ 60μm in diameter.

【Assignments】

1. Make a drawing of the transverse section of stem from Menthae Haplocalycis Herba and the microscopic characteristic drawing of the surface of leaf, show the glandular scales, non – glandular hairs, epidermal cells and stomata.

2. Make a microscopic characteristic drawing of Salviae Miltiorrhizae Radix et Rhizoma powder.

【Discussion】

1. What are the mutual macroscopic and microscopic characteristics of herbs from Labiatae Family?

2. What are the main differences of secondary structure between herbaceous stem and woody stem of dicotyledon?

实验二十四　忍冬科生药——金银花、山银花

【实验目的】

1. 掌握金银花和山银花的性状及显微鉴别特征。
2. 了解金银花和山银花的异同。

【实验指导】

忍冬科植物为灌木、乔木或藤本。多单叶，对生，少羽状复叶，常无托叶。花两性，辐射对称或两侧对称；多为聚伞花序，或再组成各种花序；花萼4~5裂；花冠管状，多5裂，有时二唇形；雄蕊与花冠裂片同数而互生，贴生于花冠管上；子房下位。浆果、核果或蒴果。本科生药以含环烯醚萜苷类和黄酮类成分为特征，并常含有绿原酸类、三萜皂苷类等成分。代表性生药有金银花、山银花等。

金银花为忍冬科植物忍冬 *Lonicera japonica* Thunb. 的干燥花蕾或带初开的花。山银花为忍冬科植物灰毡毛忍冬 *L. macranthoides* Hand. – Mazz.、红腺忍冬 *L. hypoglauca* Miq.、华南忍冬 *L. confusa* DC. 或黄褐毛忍冬 *L. fulvotomentosa* Hsu et S. C. Cheng 的干燥花蕾或带初开的花。

【仪器与试剂】

1. 仪器
光学显微镜、酒精灯、解剖针、载玻片、盖玻片等。

2. 试剂
水合氯醛溶液、稀甘油、蒸馏水等。

【实验材料】

金银花、山银花的药材标本及粉末。

【实验步骤】

1. 性状鉴别

（1）金银花

呈棒状，上粗下细，略弯曲，长2~3cm，上部直径约3mm，下部直径约1.5mm。表面黄白色或绿白色（贮久色渐深），密被短柔毛。偶见叶状苞片。花萼绿色，先端5裂，裂片有毛，长约2mm。开放者花冠筒状，先端二唇形；雄蕊5个，附于筒壁，黄色；雌蕊1个，子房无毛。气清香，味淡、微苦（图24－1）。

（2）山银花

①灰毡毛忍冬：呈棒状而稍弯曲，长3~4.5cm，上部直径约2mm，下部直径约1mm。表面黄色或黄绿色。总花梗集结成簇，开放者花冠裂片不及全长之半。质稍硬，手捏之稍有弹性。气清香，味微苦甘。

②红腺忍冬：长 2.5～4.5cm，直径 0.8～2mm。表面黄白色至黄棕色，无毛或疏被毛，萼筒无毛，先端 5 裂，裂片长三角形，被毛，开放者花冠下唇反转，花柱无毛。

③华南忍冬：长 1.6～3.5cm，直径 0.5～2mm。萼筒和花冠密被灰白色毛。

④黄褐毛忍冬：长 1～3.4cm，直径 1.5～2mm。花冠表面淡黄棕色或黄棕色，密被黄色茸毛。

2. 显微鉴别

（1）金银花

粉末浅黄棕色或黄绿色。腺毛较多，头部倒圆锥形、类圆形或略扁圆形，4～33 细胞，排成 2～4 层，直径 30～64～108μm，柄部 1～5 细胞，长可达 700μm。非腺毛有两种：一种为厚壁非腺毛，单细胞，长可达 900μm，表面有微细疣状或泡状突起，有的具螺纹；另一种为薄壁非腺毛，单细胞，甚长，弯曲或皱缩，表面有微细疣状突起。草酸钙簇晶直径 6～45μm。花粉粒类圆形或三角形，表面具细密短刺及细颗粒状雕纹，具 3 孔沟（图 24-2）。

（2）山银花

①灰毡毛忍冬：腺毛较少，头部大多圆盘形，顶端平坦或微凹，侧面观 5～16 细胞，直径 37～228μm；柄部 2～5 细胞，与头部相接处常为 2（～3）细胞并列，长 32～240μm，直径 15～51μm。厚壁非腺毛较多，单细胞，似角状，多数甚短，长 21～240（～315）μm，表面微具疣状突起，有的可见螺纹，呈短角状者体部胞腔不明显；基部稍扩大，似三角状。草酸钙簇晶，偶见。花粉粒，直径 54～82μm。

②红腺忍冬：腺毛极多，头部盾形而大，顶面观 8～40 细胞，侧面观 7～10 细胞；柄部 1～4 细胞，极短，长 5～56μm。厚壁非腺毛长短悬殊，长 38～1408μm，表面具细密疣状突起，有的胞腔内含草酸钙结晶。

③华南忍冬：腺毛较多，头部倒圆锥形或盘形，侧面观 20～60～100 细胞；柄部 2～4 细胞，长 50～176（～248）μm。厚壁非腺毛，单细胞，长 32～623（～848）μm，表面有微细疣状突起，有的具螺纹，边缘有波状角质隆起。

④黄褐毛忍冬：腺毛有两种类型：一种较长大，头部倒圆锥形或倒卵形，侧面观 12～25 细胞，柄部微弯曲，3～5（～6）细胞，长 88～470μm；另一种较短小，头部顶面观 4～10 细胞，柄部 2～5 细胞，长 24～130（～190）μm。厚壁非腺毛平直或稍弯曲，长 33～2000μm，表面疣状突起较稀，有的具菲薄横隔。

【实验报告】

1. 绘金银花和山银花粉末特征图，示腺毛、非腺毛及花粉粒。
2. 记述金银花和山银花性状区别。

【思考题】

《中国药典》自 2005 年版起，将金银花与山银花分列，其中金银花的来源为忍冬 *Lonicera japonica*，而同属多种植物的花蕾作山银花入药，《中国药典》2020 年版收载的山银花来源于灰毡毛忍冬 *L. macranthoides*、红腺忍冬 *L. hypoglauca*、华南忍冬 *L. confusa*、黄褐毛忍冬 *L. fulvotomentosa*。请结合文献查阅，分析药典变化的原因。

Experiment 24　Identification of Lonicerae Japonicae Flos and Lonicerae Flos(Caprifoliaceae)

【Objective】

1. To master the macroscopic and microscopic identification of Lonicerae Japonicae Flos and Lonicerae Flos.

2. To understand the similarities and differences between Lonicerae Japonicae Flos and Lonicerae Flos.

【Principle】

Caprifoliaceae plants are shrubs, woody climbers or small trees. Leaves mostly simple, opposite and less pinnate compound, often without stipules. Flowers bisexual, actinomorphic or bilateral; mostly cymes, or to form a variety of inflorescences; calyx 4 – or 5 – lobed; corolla tubular, much 5 – lobed, sometimes 2 – lipped; stamens and corolla lobes of the same number alternate, adnate to corolla tube; ovary inferior. Berry, drupe, or capsule. It is characterized by iridoid glycosides and flavonoids, and often contains chlorogenic acid triterpenoid saponins and other components. Representative crude drugs include Lonicerae Japonica Flos, Lonicerae Flos and so on. Lonicerae Japonica Flos is the dried bud or flower with initial blooming of *Lonicera japonica* Thunb. The Lonicera Flos is the dried flower bud or flower with initial blooming of *Lonicera macranthoides* Hand. – Mazz. , *Lonicera hypoglauca* Miq. , *Lonicera confusa* DC. or *Lonicera fulvotomentosa* Hsu et S. C. Cheng.

【Instruments and reagents】

1. Instruments
Optical microscope, alcohol lamp, anatomical needle, slide, cover glass.

2. Reagents
Chloral hydrate, dilute glycerol, distilled water.

【Materials】

Reference crude drugs of Lonicerae Japonicae Flos and Lonicerae Flos, and their powders.

【Experimental Procedures】

1. Macroscopic identification

(1) Lonicerae Japonicae Flos

Clavate, stout in upper part and tapered downwards, slightly curved, 2 ~ 3cm long, about 3mm in diameter in upper part and 1. 5mm in diameter in lower part. Externally yellowish – white or greenish – white, gradually darken on keeping, densely pubescent. Lobiform bracts occasionally visible. Calyx green,5 – lobed at the apex,lobes pubescent,about 2mm long. Corolla tubular when open,apex 2 – lipped; stamens 5,epipetalous,yellow; pistil 1,ovary glabrous. Odour delicately aromatic; taste weak and slightly bitter.

(2)Lonicerae Flos

①*Lonicera macranthoides*:Rod – shaped and slightly curved,3 ~ 4. 5cm long,with an upper diameter of about 2mm and a lower diameter of about 1mm. The surface is yellow or yellow – green. Total pedicels clustered,corolla lobes less than half full length in openers. It is slightly hard with a little elasticity in the hand. The scent is fresh and slightly bitter.

②*Lonicera hypoglauca*:2. 5 ~ 4. 5cm long,0. 8 ~ 2mm in diameter. Surface yellowish – white to yellowish – brown,glabrous or sparsely glabrous,calyx tube glabrous,apex 5 – lobed,lobed long triangular,glabrous,corolla lower lip reversed in openers,style glabrous.

③*Lonicera confuse*:1. 6 ~ 3. 5cm long,0. 5 ~ 2mm in diameter. Calyx tube and corolla densely grayish – white hairs.

④*Lonicera fulvotomentosa*:1 ~ 3. 4cm long,1. 5 ~ 2mm in diameter,the corolla surface pale yellowish – brown or yellowish – brown,densely covered with yellow hairs.

2. Microscopic identification

(1)Lonicerae Japonicae Flos

This powder is light yellowish – brown or yellowish – green. There are many glandular hairs on the head,which is conical,round or slightly oblate,with 4 ~ 33 cells arranged in 2 ~ 4 layers,30 ~ 64 ~ 108μm in diameter,1 ~ 5 cells on the stalk,up to 700μm in length. There are two types of non – glandular hairs:one is thick – walled non – glandular hair,single – celled,up to 900μm long, with tiny warts or vesicles on the surface,some with threads; the other is a thin – walled non – glandular hair,single – celled,very long,curved or wrinkled,the surface has a small vertical – like protuberance. The diameter of calcium oxalate cluster crystal is 6 ~ 45μm. Pollen grains are round or triangular in shape,with fine spines and fine grain carvings on the surface,with 3 germinal furrows.

(2)Lonicerae Flos

①*Lonicera macranthoides*:The glandular hairs are few,the head is mostly disc – shaped,the tip is flat or slightly concave,the lateral view is 5 ~ 16 cells,the diameter is 37 ~ 228μm. The stalk is 2 ~ 5 cells,often 2(~3)cells at the junction with the head,32 ~ 240μm in length and 15 ~ 51μm in diameter. Thick – walled non – glandular hairs are more,single cell,hornlike,most of them are very short,21 ~ 240(~ 315)μm long,the surface of micro vertical – like protrusions,some threads can be seen,short hornlike body cells are not obvious; base slightly enlarged,triangular – like. Calcium oxalate cluster crystals,occasionally seen. Pollen grains,54 ~ 82μm in diameter.

②*Lonicera hypoglauca*:Glandular hairs are numerous,the head is large and shield – shaped, with 8 ~ 40 cells in the apical view and 7 ~ 10 cells in the lateral view. Stalk 1 ~ 4 cells,very short, 5 ~ 56μm long. Thick – walled non – glandular hair length,long 38 ~ 1408μm,the surface with a fine vertical – like protuberance,some cells containing calcium oxalate crystal.

③*Lonicera confuse*:More glandular hairs,head inverted conical or disk – shaped,side view of 20 ~ 60 ~ 100 cells; stalk 2 ~ 4 cells,50 ~ 176(~ 248)μm long. Thick – walled non – glandular hairs, single – celled, 32 ~ 623 (~ 848) μm long, surface verrucous projections, some with threads, edge with sinuous and cuticle protuberances.

④*Lonicera fulvotomentosa*: There are two types of glandular hairs; one is larger, with an inverted conical orobovate head, 12 ~ 25 cells on the side, with a slightly curved stalk, 3 ~ 5 (~ 6) cells, with a length of 88 ~ 470μm; the other is shorter, with 4 ~ 10 cells in the apical view of the head and 2 ~ 5 cells in the stalk, 24 ~ 130 (~ 190) μm in length. Thick wall non – glandular hair straight or slightly curved, 33 ~ 2000μm long, the surface warts protrusion is relatively thin, sometimes with transverse septate.

【Assignments】

1. Draw a feature map of Lonicera Japonicae Flos and Lonicera Flos powder, showing glandular hairs, non – glandular hairs and pollen grains.

2. Record the macroscopic differences between Lonicera Japonicae Flos and Lonicera Flos.

【Discussion】

1. In the Ch. P. (2005 edition), Lonicera Japonicae Flos and Lonicera Flos have been classified separately. The source of Lonicera Japonicae Flos is the flower buds of Lonicera japonica, and the flower buds of other species from the same genus are used as medicine. The Ch. P. (2020 edition) stipulates that Lonicera Japonicae Flos is derived from *L. macranthoides*, *L. hypoglauca*, *L. confusa*, *L. fulvotomentosa*. Please review the literature and analyze the reasons for the changes in the Pharmacopoeia.

实验二十五　菊科生药——红花

【实验目的】

1. 掌握红花的性状及显微鉴别特征。
2. 熟悉菊科生药的主要鉴别方法。

【实验指导】

菊科植物多为草本；花密集成头状花序；小花异型或同型；聚药雄蕊。有香气，常具各种腺毛；有的则具有分泌道、油室；并具有各种草酸钙结晶。此外常含有菊糖。该科生药主要含有倍半萜内酯、黄酮类、生物碱、香豆素、三萜皂苷等。代表生药包括青蒿、红花、苍术、白术等。

红花为菊科植物红花 *Carthamus tinctorius* L. 的干燥花。

【仪器与试剂】

1. 仪器

光学显微镜、酒精灯、解剖针、载玻片、盖玻片等

2. 试剂

水合氯醛溶液、稀甘油、蒸馏水等。

【实验材料】

红花药材标本及粉末。

【实验步骤】

1. 性状鉴别

本品为不带子房的管状花，长 1～2cm。表面黄红色或红色。花冠筒细长，先端 5 裂，裂片狭线形；雄蕊 5 枚，花药聚合成筒状，黄白色；柱头长圆柱形，露出于花药筒外，顶端微分叉。质轻，柔软。气微香，味微苦（图 25-1）。

2. 显微鉴别

粉末橙黄色。花冠、花丝、柱头碎片多见，有长管道状分泌细胞，常位于导管旁，直径约至 66μm，含黄棕色至红棕色分泌物。花粉粒类圆形、椭圆形或橄榄形，直径约至 60μm，具 3 个萌发孔，外壁有齿状突起。草酸钙方晶存在于薄壁细胞中，直径 2～6μm。花冠裂片顶端表皮细胞外壁突起呈短绒毛状。柱头及花柱上部细胞分化成圆锥形单细胞毛，先端尖或稍钝（图 25-2）。

【实验报告】

绘红花花粉粒、柱头上的单细胞非腺毛、含色素管状分泌细胞图。

【思考题】

1. 花类生药的性状鉴别的要点有哪些?
2. 采红花应该选择什么样的天气? 为什么?

Experiment 25　Identification of Carthami Flos(Compositae)

【Objective】

1. To master the macroscopic and microscopic identification of Carthami Flos.
2. To be familiar with the method of determination of crude drugs from Compositae.

【Principle】

Compositae are mostly herbaceous; the flowers are clustered in a head; florets heteromorphic or homomorphic; synantherous stamen. Aroma, and glandular hairsvarity. Some drugs possess secretory canal and calcium oxalate crystal. In addition, it often contains inulin. The main constituents in the crude drug are sesquiterpenoids, flavonoids, alkaloids, coumarins and so on. The representative crude drugs from compositae are Artemisiae Annuae Herba, Carthami Flos, Atractylodis Rhizoma, Aucklandiae Radix and so on.

Carthami Flos is the dried flower of *Carthamus tinctorius* L. of Compositae.

【Instruments and Reagents】

1. Instruments
Optical microscope, alcohol lamp, anatomical needle, slide, cover glass.

2. Reagents
Chloral hydrate, dilute glycerin, distilled water.

【Materials】

Reference crude drug of Carthami Flos and its powder.

【Experimental Procedures】

1. Macroscopic identification
The drug consisting of tubular flowers without ovaries, 1 ~ 2cm long. Externally yellowish – red or red. Corolla tubes slender, 5 – lobe at the apex, the lobes narrowly belt – shaped. Staments 5, anthers aggregated to tube, yellowish – white. Stigma long cylindrical, slightly 2 – cleft. Texture pliable. Odour, slightly aromatic; taste, slightly bitter.

2. Microscopic identification
Powder orange – yellow. The fragments of corolla, filament and stigma frequently visible. Long

tubular secretory cells present generally accompanied by vessels up to $66\mu m$ in diameter, containing yellowish – brown to reddish – brown secretion. Pollen grains subrounded, elliptical or olivary, up to $60\mu m$ in diameter, with 3 germinal pores, exine dentate – spinose. Prisms of calcium oxalate occurring in parenchymatous cells, $2 \sim 6\mu m$ in diameter. Outer walls of terminal epidermal cells of corolla lobes projecting to be tomentellate. Upper epidermal cells of stigma and style differentiated into conical unicellular hairs, acuminate or slightly obtuse at the apex.

【Assignments】

Draw the draft of powder of Carthami Flos, including pollens, unicellular nonglandular hairs on the stigma, tubular secretory cells with pigments.

【Discussion】

1. What are the main points of macroscopic and microscopic identification of flower?
2. What kind of weather is fitting to gather Carthami Flos? Why?

实验二十六　鸢尾科生药——西红花

【实验目的】

1. 掌握西红花的性状及显微鉴别特征。
2. 熟悉西红花的与易混淆品种的鉴别方法。

【实验指导】

鸢尾科植物类为多年生草本，有根茎、块茎或鳞茎。叶常聚生茎基部。花两性，花被花瓣状。该类生药特征性化学成分为异黄酮和呫酮类。代表生药包括西红花、鸢尾等。

西红花为鸢尾科植物番红花 *Crocus sativus* L. 的干燥柱头。

【仪器与试剂】

1. 仪器

光学显微镜、酒精灯、解剖针、载玻片、盖玻片等。

2. 试剂

水合氯醛溶液、稀甘油、蒸馏水等。

【实验材料】

西红花药材标本及粉末。

【实验步骤】

1. 性状鉴别

本品呈线形，三分枝，长约3cm。暗红色，上部较宽而略扁平，顶端边缘显不整齐的齿状，内侧有一短裂隙，下端有时残留一小段黄色花柱。体轻，质松软，无油润光泽，干燥后质脆易断。气特异，微有刺激性，味微苦（图26-1）。

2. 显微鉴别

粉末橙红色。表皮细胞表面观长条形，壁薄，微弯曲，有的外壁凸出呈乳头状或绒毛状，表面隐约可见纤细纹理。柱头顶端表皮细胞绒毛状，直径26～56μm，表面有稀疏纹理。草酸钙结晶聚集于薄壁细胞中，呈颗粒状、圆簇状、梭形或类方形，直径2～14μm（图26-2）。

【实验报告】

1. 记述西红花的特征，并写出西红花和红花性状的差异。
2. 绘西红花粉末特征图。

【思考题】

如何用水试的方法区别红花和西红花？

113

Experiment 26 Identification of Croci Stigma(Iridaceae)

【Objective】

1. To master the macroscopic and microscopic identification of Croci Stigma.

2. To be familiar with the identification methods of Croci Stigma distinguishing from its confused herbal medicines.

【Principle】

Iridaceae are perennial herbs with roots, tubers or bulbs. Leaves often gather at the base of the stem. Flowers bisexual, tepals. The characteristic chemical components of this kind of crude drugs are isoflavones and kousanones. Representative herbs include Croci Stigma, Iris Tectorum Rhizoma and so on.

Croci Stigma is the dried stigma of *Crocus sativus* L. of Iridaceae.

【Instruments and Reagents】

1. Instruments

Optical microscope, alcohol lamp, anatomical needle, slide, cover glass.

2. Reagents

Chloral hydrate solution, dilute glycerin, distilled water.

【Materials】

Reference crude drug of Croci Stigma and its powder.

【Experimental Procedures】

1. Macroscopic identification

Linear, 3 – branched about 3cm long, dark red, the upper part broader and slightly flattened, the margin of apex irregularly dentate, with a short slit at the inner side, sometimes a small piece of yellow style remained at the lower end. Texture light, lax and soft, without oily luster, brittle and easily broken after drying. Odour, characteristic, slightly irritant; taste, slightly bitter.

2. Microscopic identification

Powder orange red, epidermal cells long strip – shaped in surface view, thin – walled, slightly sinuous, sometimes the outer walls protruding and showing papillae, with indistinct fine striations. Terminal epidermal cells of stigma papillated, $26 \sim 56 \mu m$ in diameter, with sparse striation on surface. Crystals of calcium embedded in parenchymatous cells, granular, round – fascicled, fusiform of subsquare, $2 \sim 14 \mu m$ in diameter. Pollen grains visible occasionally, colorless or pale yellow, spheroidal, $71 \sim 166(\sim 200) \mu m$ in diameter, exine with sparse spiny sculptures.

【Assignments】

1. Make record the characters of Croci Stigma and state the description difference between Croci Stigma and Carthami Flos.

2. Make a diagram of the characters of powder of Croci Stigma.

【Discussion】

How to distinguish Croci Stigma and Carthami Flos using water test.

实验二十七　姜科生药——砂仁

【实验目的】

1. 掌握砂仁的性状及显微鉴别特征。
2. 熟悉姜科的常用生药。

【实验指导】

姜科植物为草本，通常有芳香或辛辣味的块茎或根茎。单叶，多有叶鞘和叶舌；花两侧对称；花被片6枚，2轮。蒴果，稀浆果。本科植物多含挥发油，是化学成分的主要特征。代表性生药有砂仁、草豆蔻、干姜等。

砂仁为姜科植物阳春砂 *Amomum villosum* Lour. 、绿壳砂 *Amomum villosum* Lour. var. *xanthioides* T. L. Wu et Senjen 或海南砂 *Amomum longiligulare* T. L. Wu 的干燥成熟果实。

【仪器与试剂】

1. 仪器

光学显微镜、酒精灯、解剖针、载玻片、盖玻片等。

2. 试剂

水合氯醛溶液、稀甘油、蒸馏水等。

【实验材料】

砂仁药材标本及粉末；砂仁（阳春砂）种子横切面永久制片。

【实验步骤】

1. 性状鉴别

阳春砂呈椭圆形或卵圆形，有不明显的三棱，长 1.5~2cm，直径 1~1.5cm。表面棕褐色，密生刺状突起，顶端有花被残基，基部常有果梗。果皮薄而软。种子集结成团，具三钝棱，中有白色隔膜，将种子团分成3瓣，每瓣有种子5~26粒。种子为不规则多面体，直径 2~3mm；表面棕红色或暗褐色，有细皱纹，外被淡棕色膜质假种皮；质硬，胚乳灰白色。气芳香而浓烈，味辛凉、微苦（图 27-1）。

2. 显微鉴别

（1）阳春砂种子横切面

假种皮有时残存；种皮表皮1列，径向延长，壁稍厚；下皮细胞1列，含棕色或红棕色物；油细胞层为1列油细胞，长 76~106μm，宽 16~25μm，含黄色油滴；色素层为数列棕色细胞，细胞多角形，排列不规则；内种皮为1列栅状厚壁细胞，黄棕色，内壁及侧壁极厚，细胞小，内含硅质块；外胚乳细胞和内胚乳细胞均含淀粉粒（图 27-2）。

（2）粉末

灰棕色。内种皮厚壁细胞红棕色或黄棕色，表面观多角形，壁厚，非木化，胞腔内含硅质块；断面观为 1 列栅状细胞，内壁及侧壁极厚，胞腔偏外侧，内含硅质块。种皮表皮细胞淡黄色，表面观长条形，常与下皮细胞上下层垂直排列。下皮细胞含棕色或红棕色物。此外，尚可见色素层细胞、外胚乳和内胚乳细胞、淀粉粒、油细胞等（图 27 - 3）。

【实验报告】

绘阳春砂种子横切面组织简图和粉末显微特征图，示内种皮厚壁细胞、种皮表皮及下皮细胞。

【思考题】

1. 种子类生药的性状鉴别和显微鉴别有哪些要点？
2. 除阳春砂外，还有哪些植物的果实在部分地区作砂仁用？

Experiment 27　Identification of Amomi Fructus(Zingiberaceae)

【Objective】

1. To master the macroscopic and microscopic identification of Amomi Fructus.
2. To be familiar with common drugs from Zingiberaceae.

【Principle】

Zingiberaceae are herbaceous plants, usually having aromatic or pungent tubers or rhizomes. Leaf blade simple, with leaf sheath and leaf tongue. Flowers symmetrical on both sides; Tepals 6,2 rounds. Capsule, sparse berry. Many plants contain volatile oil, which is the main characteristic of chemical composition. Representative crude drugs are Amomi Fructus, Amomi Rotundus Fructus, Zingiberis Rhizoma and so on.

Amomi Fructus is the dried ripe fruit of *Amomum villosum* Lour. ,*Amomum villosum* Lour. var. *xanthioides* T. L. Wu et Senjen,*Amomum longiligulare* T. L. Wu of Zingiberaceae.

【Instruments and Reagents】

1. Instruments

Optical microscope, alcohol lamp

2. Reagents

Chloral hydrate, distilled water.

【Materials】

Amomi Fructus.

【Experimental Procedures】

1. Macroscopic identification

Fruit of *Amomum villosum* ellipsoidal or ovoid, indistinctly 3 – ridged, 1. 5 ~ 2cm long, 1 ~ 1. 5cm in diameter. Externally brown, densely covered with spiny protrudings, apex with remains of perianth, and base often bearing a fruit stalk. Pericarp thin and soft. Seeds agglutinated into a mass, 3 – ridged obtusely, divided into 3 groups by white septa, and each group containing 5 ~ 26 seeds. Seeds irregularly polyhedral, 2 ~ 3mm in diameter; externally brownish – red or dark brown, finely wrinkled, covered with pale brown membranous aril; texture hard, endosperm greyish – white. Odour, strongly aromatic; taste, pungent, cool and slightly bitter.

2. Microscopic identification

(1) Transverse section of seed of Fructus Amomum villosum

Sometimes remains of aril present. Epidermal cells of testa 1 row, radially elongated, slightly thick – walled; hypodermal cells 1 row, containing brown or reddish – brown contents. Oil cells in 1 row 76 ~ 100μm long, 16 ~ 25μm wide, containing yellow oil droplets. Pigment layer consisting of several rows of brown cells, polygonal, and irregularly arranged. Endotesta consisting 1 row of palisade – like thick – walled cell, yellowish – brown, small, with heavily thickened inner and lateral walls, containing a silica body. Cells of perisperm containing starch granules and a few fine prisms of calcium oxalate. Cells of endosperm containing small aleurone grains and fatty oil droplets.

(2) Powder

Greyish – brown. Thick – walled cells of endotesta reddish – brown or yellowish – brown, polygonal in surface view, with thickened and non – lignified walls, lumen containing a silica body; showing 1 row of palisade cells in section view with heavily thickened inner and lateral walls, lumen inclined to the outer side and containing a silica body. Epidermal cells of testa pale yellow, stripe – shaped in surface view, usually vertically arranged with hypodermal cells in an upper and lower layered pattern. Hypodermal cells containing brown or reddish – brown contents. Cells of pigment layer; cells of perisperm, cells of endosperm, starch grains and oil cells can be seen.

【Assignments】

Make diagrams of transverse section and powder from Amomi Fructus, and show the thick – walled cells of endotesta, epidermal cells of testa and hypodermal cells.

【Discussion】

1. What are the key points of macroscopic identification and microscopic identification for seed drugs?

2. Besides Fruit of *Amomum villosum* what other fruits of plants are used as Amomi Fructus locally?

实验二十八　兰科生药——天麻、石斛

【实验目的】

1. 掌握石斛、天麻的性状及显微鉴别特征。
2. 熟悉单子叶植物茎的主要鉴别特征。
3. 了解天麻的常见伪品与天麻在性状、显微特征上的主要区别。

【实验指导】

兰科类植物为多年生草本。花多为两性；两侧对称。蒴果。种子极多，微小粉状。主要化学成分为酚苷类、生物碱类和黏液质，并含有黄酮类、甾醇类及挥发油等。代表性生药包括天麻、石斛、白及等。

天麻为兰科植物天麻 *Gastrodia elata* Bl. 的干燥块茎。

石斛为兰科植物金钗石斛 *Dendrobium nobile* Lindl. 、霍山石斛 *Dendrobium huoshanense* C. Z. Tang et S. J. Cheng、鼓槌石斛 *Dendrobium chrysotoxum* Lindl. 或流苏石斛 *Dendrobium fimbriatum* Hook. 的栽培品及其同属植物近似种的新鲜或干燥茎。

【仪器与试剂】

1. 仪器

光学显微镜、酒精灯、解剖针、载玻片、盖玻片等。

2. 试剂

水合氯醛、蒸馏水、稀甘油等。

【实验材料】

天麻、石斛药材标本及粉末；天麻（块茎）横切面永久制片；石斛（茎）横切面永久制片。

【实验步骤】

1. 性状鉴别

（1）天麻

块茎长椭圆形，稍扁缩弯曲，长 3～15cm，宽 1.5～6cm，厚 0.5～2cm。表面黄白色至黄褐色，多不规则纵皱纹，有由潜伏芽排列成的多轮横环纹，有时可见棕黑色菌丝。顶端有红棕色鹦哥嘴状顶芽（冬麻），或残留有茎基（春麻），末端有圆脐形疤痕。质坚实，断面较平坦，黄白色或淡棕色，角质样。气微，味甘（图 28－1）。

（2）石斛

①鲜石斛：呈圆柱形或扁圆形，长约 30cm，直径 0.4～1.2cm。表面黄绿色，光滑或有纵纹，节明显，色较深，节上有膜质叶鞘。肉质多汁，易折断。气微，味微苦而回甜，嚼之有黏性。

119

②金钗石斛：呈扁圆柱形，长 20 ~ 40cm，直径 0.4 ~ 0.6cm，节间长 2.5 ~ 3cm。表面金黄色或黄中带绿色，有深纵沟。质硬而脆，断面较平坦而疏松。气微，味苦。

③鼓槌石斛：呈粗纺锤形，中部直径 1 ~ 3cm，具 3 ~ 7 节。表面光滑，金黄色，有明显凸起的棱。质轻而松脆，断面海绵状。气微，味淡，嚼之有黏性。

④流苏石斛：呈长圆柱形，长 20 ~ 150cm，直径 0.4 ~ 1.2cm，节明显，节间长 2 ~ 6cm。表面黄色至暗黄色，有深纵槽。质疏松，断面平坦或呈纤维性。味淡或微苦，嚼之有黏性（图 28 - 2）。

2. 显微鉴别

（1）天麻

①天麻块茎横切面：表皮有时残存；下皮为 2 ~ 3 列切向延长的木栓化细胞。皮层为 10 数列多角形细胞，有的含草酸钙针晶束。较老块茎外侧皮层为 2 ~ 3 列厚壁细胞，壁木化，有纹孔。中柱大，周韧型维管束散列；薄壁细胞含草酸钙针晶束（图 28 - 3，图 28 - 4，图 28 - 5）。

②粉末：粉末黄白色至黄棕色。厚壁细胞椭圆形或类多角形，直径 70 ~ 180μm，壁厚 3 ~ 8μm，木化，纹孔明显。草酸钙针晶成束或散在，长 25 ~ 75（93）μm。用甘油醋酸试液装片观察含糊化多糖类物的薄壁细胞无色，有的细胞可见长卵形、长椭圆形或类圆形颗粒，遇碘液显棕色或淡棕紫色。螺纹导管、网纹导管及环纹导管直径 8 ~ 30μm（图 28 - 6）。

（2）石斛

①金钗石斛茎横切面：扁圆形，边缘有 6 ~ 7 个浅波。表皮为 1 列细小扁平细胞，外被厚的角质层。基本薄壁组织中散列多数有限外韧型维管束，略成 7 ~ 8 圈；维管束外侧有半月形纤维束，1 ~ 4 列，其外缘嵌有细小薄壁细胞，有的含圆簇状硅质块；木质部有 1 ~ 3 个导管较大。黏液细胞含草酸钙针晶束，长 50 ~ 130μm（图 28 - 7，图 28 - 8）。

②粉末：灰绿色或灰黄色。角质层碎片黄色；表皮细胞表面观呈长多角形或类多角形，垂周壁连珠状增厚。束鞘纤维成束或离散，长梭形或细长，壁较厚，纹孔稀少，周围具排成纵行的含硅质块的小细胞。木纤维细长，末端尖或钝圆，壁稍厚。网纹导管、梯纹导管或具缘纹孔导管直径 12 ~ 50μm。草酸钙针晶成束或散在（图 28 - 9）。

【实验报告】

1. 列表记述石斛类生药的组织特征鉴别要点，并绘金钗石斛茎横切面简图。

2. 绘石斛粉末特征图，示晶鞘纤维、表皮细胞。

3. 绘天麻块茎横切面组织简图。

4. 绘天麻粉末特征图，示厚壁细胞、草酸钙针晶束、多糖团块。

【思考题】

1. 天麻的伪品有哪些？

2. 如何从性状上区别上述 5 种石斛？

Experiment 28　Identification of Gastrodiae Rhizoma and Dendrobii Caulis(Orchidaceae)

【Objective】

1. To master the macroscopic and microscopic identification of Gastrodiae Rhizoma and Dendrobii Caulis.

2. To be familiar with the main distinguishing characters of stems from Monocotyledoneae.

3. To understandthe distinguishing characters of *Gastrodia elata* and its adulterants

【Principle】

Orchidaceae are perennial herbs. Flowers are mostly bisexual; Bilateral symmetry. Capsule. The seeds are numerous and tiny, powdery. The main chemical components are phenolic glycosides. Alkaloids and slime, and contains flavonoids, sterols and volatile oil, etc. Representative crude drugs include Gastrodiae, Rhizoma, Dendrobil Caulis, Bletillae Rhizoma.

Gastrodiae Rhizoma is the dried tuber of *Gastrodia elata* Bl. of Orchidaceae.

Dendrobii Caulis is the fresh or dried stem of *Dendrobium nobile* Lindl. , *Dendrobium huoshanense* C. Z. Tang et S. J. Cheng, *Dendrobium chrysotoxum* Lindl. , *Dendrobium fimbriatum* Hook. or their cultivating and allied species of Orchidaceae.

【Instruments and Reagents】

1. Instruments
Optical microscope, alcohol lamp, anatomical needle, slide, cover glass.

2. Reagents
Chloral hydrate, dilute glycerin, distilled water.

【Materials】

Reference crude drugs of Gastrodiae Rhizoma and Dendrobii Caulis, and their powders; sildes of tuber transverse section of *Gastrodia elata*; sildes of stem transverse section of *Dendrobium nobile*.

【Experimental Procedures】

1. Macroscopic identification

(1)Gastrodiae Rhizoma

Ellipsoid or slat – shaped, slightly compressed, shrunken and somewhat curved, 3 ~ 15cm long, 1. 5 ~ 6cm wide, 0. 5 ~ 2cm thick. Externally yellowish – white to yellowish – brown, with longitudinal wrinkles and many transverse annulations arranged by latent buds, sometimes brown funiculi visible. Apex with reddish – brown to deep brown parrot – beak – like buds or remains of stem, the lower end with a rounded scar. Texture hard and uneasily broken, fracture fairly even, yellowish – white to brownish, horny. Odour, slight; taste, sweetish.

(2) Dendrobii Caulis

①Fresh Dendrobium：Cylindrical or flattened – cylindrical, about 30cm long, 0. 4 ~ 1. 2cm in diameter. Externally yellowish – green, smooth or striated longitudinally, with distinct nodes, deeply colored, bearing membranous leaf sheaths. Fleshy, succulent, easily broken. Odour slight; taste slightly bitter, then sweet and viscous on chewing.

②Stem of *D. nobile*：Flattened – cylindrical, 20 ~ 40cm long, 4 ~ 6mm diameter, internodes 2. 5 ~ 3cm long. Externally golden or greenish – yellow, deeply furrowed longitudinally. Texture hard and fragile, fracture relatively even and lax, odour slight; taste bitter.

③Stem of *D. chrysotoxum*：Thickspidle – shaped, 1 ~ 3cm in diameter in middle part, with 3 ~ 7 nodes. Externally smooth, golden, longitudinally angular convex distinct. Texture light, lax and fragile, fracture spongy. Odour slight; taste weak and viscous on chewing.

④Stem of *D. fimbriatum* and the other similar species：Long cylindrical, 20 ~ 150cm long, 0. 4 ~ 1. 2cm in diameter, with distinct nodes, internodes 2 ~ 6cm long. Externally yellow to dark yellow, deeply furrowed longitudinally. Texture lax, fracture even or fibrous. Taste weak or slightly bitter, viscous on chewing.

2. Microscopic identification

(1) Gastrodiae Rhizoma

①Transverse isection：Remains of epidermis present, hypodermis of 2 ~ 3 rows of suberized and tangentially elongated cells. Cortex consisting of over 10 rows of polygonal cells, some containing raphides of calcium oxalate. In older tubers 2 ~ 3 rows of elliptical sclerenchymatous cells present in cortex adjacent to hypodermis, with lignified and obviously pitted walls. Stele occupied the most part of rhizome, scattered small amphicribral vascular bundles, parenchymatous cells containing raphides of calcium oxalate.

②Powder：Yellowish – white to yellowish brown. Sclerenchymatous cells elliptical or subpolygonal, 70 ~ 180μm in diameter, walls 3 ~ 8μm in thickness, lignified, distinctly, pitted. Needle crystals of calcium oxalate in bundles or scattered, 25 ~ 75 (93) μm long. When mounted in glycerin – acetic acid TS, parenchymatous cells containing gelatinized polysaccharides colorless, and some cells containing long – ovoid, long – ellipsoid or subrounded granules, showing a brown or brownish – purple color on adding iodine solution. Spiral, reticulated and annual vessels 8 ~ 30μm in diameter.

(2) Dendrobii Caulis

①Transverse section of Stem of *D. nobile*：Flattened – rounded, 6 ~ 7 shallow waves on the edge. Epidermal cells of 1 layer small and flattened, covered with thick cuticle. Basic parenchymatous tissues, scattered with numerous closed collateral vascular bundles, somewhat arranged in 7 ~ 8 whorls; fibre bundles at the outer side of vascular bundles crescent or semicircular, 1 ~ 4 layers, small parenchymatous cells at the outer side part containing subrounded silica bodies; xylem with 1 ~ 3 relatively large vessels. Mucus cells containing needle crystal bundles of calcium oxalate, 50 ~ 130μm long.

②Powder：Fibres outside of vascular bundles mostly in bundles or scattered, long – shuttled, cells around fiber bundles containing subrounded silica bodies, arranged in rows longitudinally. Needle crystal bundles of calcium oxalate occurring in parenchymatous cells, needle crystals relatively thick. Epidermal cells in surface view long – polygon, anticlinal walls beaded thickened, chicken wire cracking on the surface of cuticle. Woody fibre mostly in bundles, pits more, with small bordered pits.

【Assignments】

1. List the key points for identification of tissue characteristics of dendrobium crude drugs. Make a drawing of transverse section of Gastrodiae Rhizoma.

2. Draw characteristic drawings of the powder of Dendrobii Caulis, and signify the crystal fibres, epidermal cells.

3. Draw the diagram of the transverse section of Gastrodiae Rhizoma.

4. Make a diagnostic drawing of powder of Gastrodiae Rhizoma, and signify the sclerenchymatous cells, raphides of calcium oxalate and amylose conglomeration.

【Discussion】

1. What are the adulterants of Gastrodiae Rhizoma?

2. How to distinct the mentioned five kinds of crude drugs from Genus *Dendrobium* by macroscopic identification?

实验二十九　动物类生药——斑蝥、全蝎

【实验目的】

1. 掌握斑蝥、全蝎的性状及显微鉴别特征。
2. 了解节肢动物体壁的构造及显微鉴别要点。

【实验指导】

动物类生药显微特征包括动物的组织，如横纹肌、体壁碎片、刚毛、骨碎片等。另外某些动物部分需要做组织切片或磨片，如贝壳类、角类、骨类、珍珠等。动物类生药主要含有氨基酸、甾体类、生物碱类及萜类等成分。代表生药包括鹿茸、全蝎、斑蝥、牛黄等。

斑蝥为芫青科昆虫南方大斑蝥 *Mylabri sphalerata* Pallas 或黄黑小斑蝥 *Mylabris cichorii* Linnaeus 的干燥体。

全蝎为钳蝎科动物东亚钳蝎 *Buthus martensii* Karsch 的干燥体。

【仪器与试剂】

1. 仪器
光学显微镜、酒精灯、解剖针、载玻片、盖玻片等。

2. 试剂
水合氯醛溶液、稀甘油、蒸馏水等。

【实验材料】

斑蝥、全蝎。

【实验步骤】

1. 性状鉴别

（1）斑蝥

①南方大斑蝥：虫体呈长圆形，长 1.5~2.5cm，宽 0.5~1cm，头及口器下垂，有较大的复眼及触角各 1 对，触角多已脱落。背部具革质鞘翅 1 对，黑色，有黄色或棕黄色横纹 3 条，鞘翅下有棕色膜状透明的内翅 2 片。胸腹部乌黑色，有光泽，胸部有足 3 对。有特殊异臭。

②黄黑小斑蝥：体型较小，长 1~1.5cm（图 29-1）。

（2）全蝎

本品头胸部与前腹部呈扁平长椭圆形，后腹部呈尾状，皱缩弯曲，完整者体长约 6cm。头胸部呈绿褐色，前面有 1 对短小的螯肢和 1 对较长大的钳状脚须，形似蟹螯，背面覆有梯形背甲，腹面有足 4 对，均为 7 节，末端各具 2 爪钩；前腹部由 7 节组成，第 7 节色深，背甲上有 5 条隆脊线。背面绿褐色，后腹部棕黄色，6 节，节上均有纵沟，末节有锐钩状毒刺，毒刺下方无距。气微腥，味咸（图 29-2）。

2. 显微鉴别

（1）斑蝥

本品粉末棕褐色。

①体壁碎片黄白色至棕褐色，表面隐见斜向纹理，可见短小的刺、刚毛或刚毛脱落后留下的凹窝。

②刚毛多碎断，棕褐色或棕红色，完整者平直或呈镰刀状弯曲，先端锐尖；表面可见斜向纵纹。

③横纹肌纤维碎块近无色或淡黄棕色，表面可有明暗相间的波状纹理；侧面观常数条成束，表面淡黄棕色或黄白色，可见顺直纹理。

④鞘翅碎片淡棕黄色或棕红色，角质不规则形，表面有稀疏刚毛及凹陷的圆形环，直径28~120μm。

⑤气管壁碎片不规则，条状增厚壁呈棕色或深棕色螺旋状（图29-3）。

（2）全蝎

①体壁碎片外表皮表面观呈多角形网格样纹理，表面密布细小颗粒，可见毛窝、细小圆孔和淡棕色或近无色的瘤状突起；内表皮无色，有横向条纹，内、外表皮纵贯较多长短不一的微细孔道。

②刚毛红棕色，多碎断，先端锐尖或钝圆，具纵直纹理，髓腔细窄。

③横纹肌纤维多碎断，明带较暗带宽，明带中有一暗线，暗带有致密的短纵纹理（图29-4）。

【实验报告】

1. 描述全蝎体壁碎片、刚毛及横纹肌纤维三者的鉴别要点。

2. 绘全蝎体壁表面观和刚毛的显微鉴别特征图。

【思考题】

如何鉴别斑蝥和青娘子，两者在功效上有何不同？

Experiment 29　Identification of Mylabris and Scorpio

【Objective】

1. To master the macroscopic and microscopic identification of Mylabris and Scorpio.

2. To understand the structure of body walls and microscopical differential points of arthropods.

【Principle】

The microscopic characteristics of the crude drug from animals: segment of voluntary muscle, integument, bristles, bone chips and so on. Tissue biopsies or slice were needed for some drugs, such as shells, horns, bones and pearls. The main constituents in the crude drug are amino acids, alkaloids, terpenoids, steroids and so on. The important drugs from animals contains Cervi Cornu

Pantotrichunm, Scorpio, Mylabris, Bovis Calculus and so on.

Mylabris is the dried body of *Mylabris phalerata* Pallas or *Mylabris cichorii* Linnaeus of Meloidae.

Scorpio is the dried body of *Buthus martensii* Karsch of Buthidae.

【Instruments and Reagents】

1. Instruments

Optical microscope, alcohol lamp, anatomical needle, slide, cover glass.

2. Reagents

Chloral hydrate, dilute glycerin, distilled water.

【Materials】

Reference crude drugs of Mylabris and Scorpio and their powders.

【Experimental Procedures】

1. Macroscopic identification

(1) Mylabris

①Body of *Mylabris phalerata*: Body elongated round, 1.5 ~ 2.5cm long, 0.5 ~ 1cm wide, the head and the mouth parts curved downward, with a pair of relatively large compound eyes and a pair of antennae which usually fallen off. A pair of leathery elytra on the dorsum, black, with three yellow or brownish - yellow transverse stripes, a pair of transparent brownish membrane - like hind wings beneath the elytra. The thorax and abdomen pitch - black, with three pairs of legs at the thorax. Odour characteristic stinking.

②Body of *Mylabris cichorii*: Body size relatively small, 1 ~ 1.5cm long.

(2) Scorpio

The cehalothorax and preabdomen flattened long ellipsoidal, the postabdomen tail - like, shrunken and curved, the body of intact specimen about 6cm long. The cephalothorax greenish - brown, the anterior part arising 1 pair of short and small chelicerae and 1 pair of long and large pincerlike pedipalps in the shape of crab pincers, dorsal part bearing 4 pairs of walking legs, each of segments, with 2 claws on distal end. The preabdomen consist of 7 segments, the seventh dark in color, with 5 ridged spinal lines on the dorsal plate. Dorsal side greenish - brown, the postabdomen brownish - yellow, 6 segments, with longitudinal furrows on each segment, the telson bearing sharp claw like stinger and no spur below the stinger. Odour, slightly stinking; taste, salty.

2. Microscopic identification

(1) Mylabris

Fragments of body walls yellowish - white or brown, reticulate striations in surface view, fine rounded holes and pale brown or nearly colorless tumor protrusions visible. Setae brown or redish - brown, mostly broken. The complete seta is sickle - shaped. Striped muscle fibers mostly broken, the bright strips broader than the dark ones, each bright strip of a dark thread, dark strip with dense short longitudinal striations. Fragments of elytrum redish - brown or yellowish - brown, incomplete, fine rounded holes and pale brown or nearly colorless tumor protrusions visible. The fragments of trachea irregular, spiral and brown.

（2）Scorpio

Fragments of body wallschitinized, lustrous; epidermis showing polygonal reticulate striations in surface view, surface densely covered with minute granules, setae pits, fine rounded holes and pale brown or nearly colorless tumor protrusions visible; outer surface greenish – yellow and inner surface colorless in cross section view, transverse striations visible, many long or short porous channels penetrating across the epidermis and endodermis. Setae yellowish – brown, mostly broken, apex cuspidate or obtuse, with longitudinal straight striations, medullary cavities narrow. Striped muscle fibers mostly broken, the bright strips broader than the dark ones, each bright strip of a dark thread, dark strip with dense short longitudinal striations.

【Assignments】

1. Describe the microscopical points of fragments of body walls, setae and striped muscle fibers from Scorpio.

2. Draw the characteristic diagrams of body walls（in surface view）and setae of Scorpio.

【Discussion】

How to identify Cylabris and Lytta Caraganae Pallas? What are the differences between the two in action?

实验三十　动物类生药——珍珠、牡蛎

【实验目的】

1. 掌握珍珠、牡蛎性状及显微鉴别特征。
2. 了解常用的海洋类生药。

【实验指导】

海洋来源的动物类生药种类众多，性状及显微特征多样。该类生药主要成分包括无机物大环内酯类、肽类、聚醚类、萜类及甾体类成分。重要的生药包括牡蛎、珍珠、海马、海龙等。

珍珠为珍珠贝科动物马氏珍珠贝 *Pteria martensii*（Dunker）、蚌科动物三角帆蚌 *Hyriopsis cumingii*（*Lea.*）或褶纹冠蚌 *Cristariaplicata*（*Leach*）等双壳类动物受刺激形成的珍珠。

牡蛎为牡蛎科动物长牡蛎 *Ostrea gigas* Thunberg、大连湾牡蛎 *Ostrea talienwhanensis* Crosse 或近江牡蛎 *Ostrea rivularis* Gould 的贝壳。

【仪器与试剂】

1. 仪器
光学显微镜、酒精灯、解剖针、载玻片、盖玻片等。

2. 试剂
水合氯醛溶液、稀甘油、蒸馏水等。

【实验材料】

珍珠、牡蛎药材标本及粉末。

【实验步骤】

1. 性状鉴别

（1）珍珠

本品呈类球形、长圆形、卵圆形或棒形，直径 1.5~8mm。表面类白色、浅粉红色、浅黄绿色或浅蓝色，半透明，光滑或微有凹凸，具特有的彩色光泽。质坚硬，破碎面显层纹。气微，味淡（图 30-1）。

（2）牡蛎

①长牡蛎：呈长片状，背腹缘几平行，长 10~50cm，高 4~15cm。右壳较小，鳞片坚厚，层状或层纹状排列。壳外面平坦或具数个凹陷，淡紫色、灰白色或黄褐色；内面瓷白色，壳顶二侧无小齿。左壳凹陷深，鳞片较右壳粗大，壳顶附着面小。质硬，断面层状，洁白。气微，味微咸。

②大连湾牡蛎：呈类三角形，背腹缘呈八字形。右壳外面淡黄色，具疏松的同心鳞片，鳞片起伏成波浪状，内面白色。左壳同心鳞片坚厚，自壳顶部放射肋数个，明显，内面凹

下呈盒状，铰合面小（图 30 – 2A）。

③近江牡蛎：呈圆形、卵圆形或三角形等。右壳外面稍不平，有灰、紫、棕、黄等色，环生同心鳞片，幼体者鳞片薄而脆，多年生长后鳞片层层相叠，内面白色，边缘有的淡紫色（图 30 – 2B）。

2. 显微鉴别

（1）珍珠

本品粉末类白色。不规则碎块，半透明，具彩虹样光泽。表面显颗粒性，由数至十数薄层重叠，片层结构排列紧密，可见致密的成层线条或极细密的微波状纹理。本品磨片具同心层纹（图 30 – 3）。

（2）牡蛎

本品粉末灰白色。珍珠层呈不规则碎块，较大碎块呈条状或片状，表面隐约可见细小条纹。棱柱层少见，断面观呈棱柱状，断端平截，长 29 ~ 130 μm；宽 10 ~ 36 μm，有的一端渐尖，亦可见数个并列成排；表面观呈类多角形、方形或三角形（图 30 – 4）。

【实验报告】

1. 绘珍珠不规则碎块图。

2. 绘牡蛎不规则碎块图，包括珍珠层和棱柱层。

【思考题】

珍珠的传统真伪鉴别方式有哪些？

Experiment 30　Identification of Margarita and Ostreae Concha

【Objective】

1. To master the macroscopic and microscopic identification of Margarita and Ostreae Concha.

2. To understand the commonly used crude durgs from marine.

【Principle】

The crude drugs from marine are numerous, and morphological diversity. The main constituents in the crude drug are inorganic substance, macrolides, peptides, polyethers, terpenoids and so on. The important drugs contains Margartia, Ostreae Concha, Hippocampus.

Margarita is the peal of *Pteria martensii* (Dunker) of Pteriidae and *Hyriopsis cumingii* (Lea.) or *Cristaria plicata* (Leach) of Unionidae.

Ostreae Concha is the shell of *Ostrea gigas* Thunberg, *Ostrea talienwhanensis* Crosse, *Ostrea rivularis* Gould of Ostreidae.

【Instruments and Reagents】

1. Instruments

Optical microscope, alcohol lamp, anatomical needle, slide, cover glass.

2. Reagents

Chloral hydrate , dilute glycerin, distilled water.

【Materials】

Reference crude drugs of Margarita and Ostreae Concha, and their powders.

【Experimental Procedures】

1. Macroscopic identification

（1）Margarita

Subspheroidal, oblong, ovoid or clavate, 1. 5 ~ 8mm in diameter. Externally whitish, light pink, light yellowish – green or light blue, translucent, smooth or slightly uneven with characteristic lustre. Texture hard, laminating veins on broken surface. Odour, slight; tasteless.

（2）Ostreae Concha

①Shell of Ostrea gigas: In elongated pieces, dorsal and ventral edges almost parallel, 10 ~ 50cm long, 4 ~ 15cm high. The right shell relatively small, scales strong and thick, arranged in layers or striated. The outer surface smooth or with several depressioms, pale purple, greyish – white or yellowish – brown; the inner surface porcelain white, without denticles at both sides of the umbo. The left shell deeply depressed, scales bigger and more rough than those of the right shell, attachment surface of the umbo small. Texture hard, fracture stratiform, white. Odour, slight; taste, slight salty.

②Shell of Ostrea talienwhanensis: Subtriangular, dorsal and ventral edges V – shape. The outer surface of the right shell pale yellow, concentric scales arranged loosely and undulated up and down; the inner surface white. The left shell bearing strong and thick concentric scales, several distinct ribs radiated from the umbo, the inner surface concaved in boxshaped; hinge surface small.

③Shell of Ostrea rivularis: Rounded, oval or triangular. The outer surface of right shell slightly uneven, grey, purple, brown, yellow, etc. ; concentric scales in a ring, thin and fragile when immature and overlapped one another after several years' growth. The inner surface white, sometimes the edge pale purple.

2. Microscopic identification

（1）Margarita

Irregular pieces, translucent, with rainbow – like lustre. Surface granular, piled up by several to ten thin layers, laminae densely arranged, dense laminated lines or finely undulated striation visible. Ground slices marked with concentric striations.

（2）Ostreae Concha

Greyish – white. Nacreous layers in irregular broken pieces, big pieces strip – like or sheet – like, surface slightly finely striated. Prismatic layers visible occasionally, section view prismatic, the broken ends truncate, 29 ~ 130μm long and 10 ~ 36μm wide, some with tapering ends; surface view polygonal, square or triangle.

【Assignments】

1. Draw the draft of powder of Margarita, including irregular pieces.
2. Draw the draft of powder of Ostreae Concha, including nacreous layers and prismatic layers.

【Discussion】

How to identify Margarita byusing traditional methods?

实验三十一 矿物类生药——朱砂、雄黄

【实验目的】

1. 掌握朱砂、雄黄的组成及其性状特征。
2. 熟悉矿物类生药的理化鉴别方法。

【实验指导】

矿物药是一类特殊的生药，一般根据矿物的性质进行鉴定。对于性状鉴定，可根据外形、颜色、质地、气味、硬度、条痕、解理等进行鉴定。显微鉴定可运用显微镜观察其形状、透明度颜色等。理化鉴定主要对其化学成分进行定性定量分析。

朱砂（硫化物类矿物辰砂族辰砂，主含硫化汞），雄黄（硫化物类矿物雄黄族雄黄，主含二硫化二砷）。

【仪器与试剂】

1. 仪器
水浴锅、坩埚、烧杯、试管、铜片等。

2. 试剂
盐酸、硝酸、氯酸钾、氯化钡、硫化氢、碳酸铵、蒸馏水等。

【实验材料】

朱砂、雄黄药材标本及粉末。

【实验步骤】

1. 性状鉴别

（1）朱砂

本品为粒状或块状集合体，呈颗粒状或块片状。鲜红色或暗红色，条痕红色至褐红色，具光泽。体重，质脆，片状者易破碎，粉末状者有闪烁的光泽。气微，味淡（图31-1）。

（2）雄黄

本品为块状或粒状集合体，呈不规则块状。深红色或橙红色，条痕淡橘红色，晶面有金刚石样光泽。质脆，易碎，断面具树脂样光泽。微有特异的臭气，味淡。精矿粉为粉末状或粉末集合体，质松脆，手捏即成粉，橙黄色，无光泽（图31-2）。

2. 理化鉴别

（1）朱砂

①取本品粉末，用盐酸湿润后，在光洁的铜片上摩擦，铜片表面显银白色光泽，加热烘烤后，银白色即消失。

②取本品粉末2g，加盐酸-硝酸（3∶1）的混合溶液2ml使溶解，蒸干，加水2ml使溶解，滤过，滤液显汞盐与硫酸盐的鉴别反应。

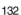

（2）雄黄

①取本品粉末 10mg，加水润湿后，加氯酸钾饱和的硝酸溶液 2ml，溶解后，加氯化钡试液，生成大量白色沉淀。放置后，倾出上层酸液，再加水 2ml，振摇，沉淀不溶解。

②取本品粉末 0.2g，置坩埚内，加热熔融，产生白色或黄白色火焰，并伴有白色浓烟。取玻片覆盖后，有白色冷凝物，刮取少量，置试管内加水煮沸使溶解，必要时滤过，溶液加硫化氢试液数滴，即显黄色，加稀盐酸后生成黄色絮状沉淀，再加碳酸铵试液，沉淀复溶解。

【实验报告】

1. 描述朱砂及雄黄的性状特征。
2. 描述朱砂及雄黄的理化鉴别特征。

【思考题】

1. 矿物类生药的硬度如何确定？
2. 什么是矿物类生药的本色、外色、假色、条痕色？

Experiment 31　Identification of Cinnabaris and Realgar

【Objective】

1. To master the morphologic identification of Cinnabaris and Realgar.

2. To be familiar with the physico – chemical identification method of mineral drugs.

【Principle】

Mineral drugs are a particular class of crude drugs, and identified by the characters of mineral. Mineral drugs could be identified by their shape, color, odour, hardness, streak and so on. We also could identify their shape and diaphaneity by microscope. Physico – chemical identification is used to analyze the chemical constitution of the mineral drugs.

Cinnabaris is from the Cinnabar family of Sulphide mineral, mainly containing HgS; Realgar is from the Realgar family of Sulphide mineral, mainly containing AS_2S_2.

【Instruments and Reagents】

1. Instruments

Water bath pot, crucible, beaker, test tube, copper sheet

2. Reagents

Hydrochloric acid, nitric acid, potassium chlorate, barium chloride, hydrogen sulfide, ammonium carbonate, distilled water.

【Materials】

Reference crude drugs of Cinnabaris and Realgar and their powders.

【Experimental Procedures】

1. Morphologic identification

（1）Cinnabaris

Aggregates of granulous or lumpy masses, in granules or pieces, bright red or dark red, streak red to brownish – red, lustrous. Texture heavy and fragile. Pieces easily broken and granules with glittering gloss. Odourless and tasteless.

（2）Realgar

Aggregates of lumpy or granulous masses, irregular, dark red or orange – red; pale orange – red streak; crystal surface showing diamond – like lustre. Texture fragile, easily broken, fracture with resin – like lustre. Odour, slightly stinking and tasteless.

Powder refined ore: In powders or powder aggregates. Texture lax and fragile, powdered on kneading. Orange – yellow, lustreless.

2. Physiochemical identification

（1）Cinnabaris

① Take the powder, wet it with hydrochloric acid, then rub it on the smooth copper sheet, the surface of the copper sheet shows silver – white luster, then the silver – white will disappear after heating and baking.

②Take 2g powder, add 2ml the mixture of hydrochloric and acidnitric acid（3:1）to dissolve it, steam dried, then add 2ml of water to dissolve, filter, filtrate to show the identification reaction of mercury salt and sulfate.

（2）Realgar

①Take 10mg powder, wet with water, then add 2ml of potassium chlorate saturated nitric acid solution to dissolve, and add barium chloride test solution, generate a large amount of white precipitation after placing. Then pour out the upper, add another 2ml of water, shake and the precipitation is not dissolved.

②Take 0.2g powder to the crucible, heating to produce white or yellowish – white flame, accompanied by a white smoke. Then take a small amount of white condensate with boilling water dissolved in a test tube and filter when necessary, and drops of hydrogen sulfide test solution showed yellow, then yellow flocculent precipitate was generated after adding dilute hydrochloric acid, and ammonium carbonate test solution was added to precipitate and redissolve.

【Assignments】

1. Describe the morphological feature of Cinnabaris and Realgar.

2. Describe the physico – chemical feature of Cinnabaris and Realgar.

【Discussion】

1. How to determine the hardness level of mineral drugs?

2. What are the intricate colour, exo – colour, false colour and streak colour of mineral drugs?

第三篇 设计性与综合性实验

Chapter Three Designable and Comprehensive Experiments

实验三十二 几种未知生药混合粉末的显微及理化鉴别

【实验目的】

1. 通过显微及理化方法掌握几种未知生药粉末的鉴别方法。

【实验指导】

1. 制作粉末临时装片，在显微镜下观察组织和细胞特性。
2. 用化学方法和物理方法对粉末中的某些成分进行检测。

实验流程如图 32 −1 所示。

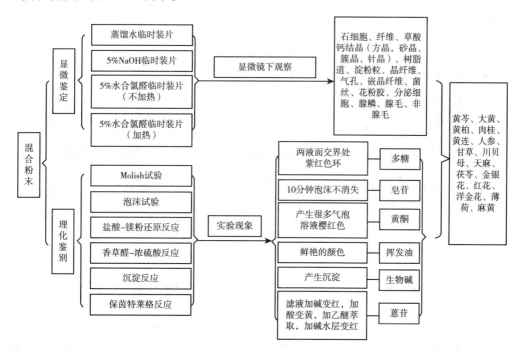

图 32 −1 混合粉末显微及理化鉴定流程

【仪器与试剂】

1. 仪器

光学显微镜、酒精灯、水浴锅、索氏提取器、薄层板、展开缸、层析滤纸等。

2. 试剂

乙醇、乙醚、三氯甲烷、水合氯醛、正丁醇、甘油、甲醇、浓盐酸、浓氨水、草酸、醋酸、醋酸铅、碘化汞钾、碘化铋钾、碘-碘化钾试液、硫酸、镁粉、蒸馏水、α-萘酚试液、Dragendorff 试剂等。

【实验材料】

黄芩、大黄、黄柏、肉桂、黄连、人参、甘草、川贝母、天麻、茯苓、金银花、红花、洋金花、薄荷、麻黄药材粉末。

【实验步骤】

1. 取粉末适量（约半粒大米粒大小）置在载玻片上，滴加甘油醋酸试液、水合氯醛试液或其他试液，盖上盖玻片。置显微镜下观察。

2. 通过物理或化学的方法，根据化学试剂与生药中的化学成分产生特殊的颜色或沉淀，对它们进行定性分析。

【实验报告】

1. 记录鉴别操作和结果。

2. 绘制显微鉴别特征图。

3. 观察并记录各类成分的反应现象。

【思考题】

1. 粉末显微鉴别临时装片时应注意哪些问题？

2. 生药的理化鉴别方法有哪些？

3. 如何鉴别含生物碱、黄酮苷、皂苷、强心苷的药材？

Experiment 32　Microscopical Identification and Physico - chemical Identification of Unknown Cude Drugs

【Objective】

1. To identify several unknown crude drugs powder by microscopic, physical and chemical methods.

【Principle】

1. Observe the characters of tissues and cells in powders under the microscope by making slides.

2. Test some constituents in the powders of crude drugs by chemical and physical methods.

The thought of the research is shown in Figure 32 - 1.

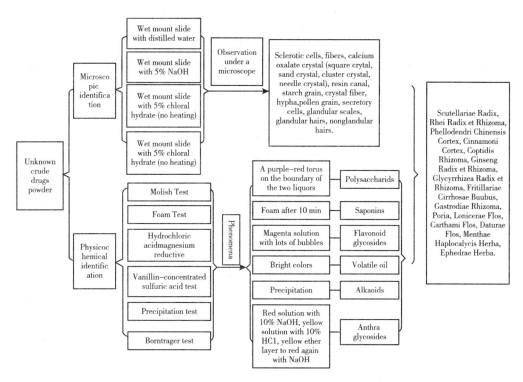

Figure 32 – 1   The diagram of the crude drugs' identification

【Instruments and Reagents】

1. Instruments

Optical microscope, alcohol lamp, water bath, Soxhlet's instruments, frosting flask, thin layer plates, saturated chamber.

2. Reagents

Ethanol, ethyl ether, chloroform, chloral hydrate, n – butanol, glycerin, methanol, concentrated hydrochloric acid, concentrated ammonia, oxalic acid, acetic acid, lead acetate, potassium mercury iodide, potassium bismuth iodide, iodide potassium test solution, sulfuric acid, magnesium powder, distilled water, α – naphthol test solution, Dragendorff reagent, etc.

【Materials】

Drug powder: Scutellariae Radix, Rhei Radix et Rhizoma, Phellodendri Chinensis Cortex, Cinnamomi Cortex, Coptidis Rhizoma, Ginseng Radix et Rhizoma, Glycyrrhizae Radix et Rhizoma, Fritillariae Cirrhosae Bulbus, Gastrodiae Rhizoma, Poria, Lonicerae Flos, Carthami Flos, Daturae Flos, Menthae Haplocalycis Herba, Ephedrae Herba.

【Procedures Experimental】

Choose several powders above at random, identify by microscopic, physical and chemical methods.

1. Spread a small quantity of the powder on a slide, and examine after treated with glycerol – acetic acid test solutions, chloral hydrate, or other suitable test solutions, and then cover with

coverslip. Observe under the optical microscope.

2. Qualitative analysis can be carried out to identify which kinds of chemical constituents are contained in crude drugs by using some chemical reagents to produce special color or sediment, which can be used to discern the fake from the genuine.

【Assignments】

1. Record the identification operations and the results of crude drugs.

2. Draw the diagrams of microscopic identification characteristics.

3. Observe and record the reaction phenomenon of various constituents.

【Discussion】

1. What should be paid attention to the slide of powder in microscopic identification of the crude drugs?

2. What are the physico – chemical identification methods of the crude drugs?

3. How to identify the crude drugs containing alkaloids, flavonoid glycosides, saponins, or cardiac glycosides?

实验三十三　位点特异性 PCR 法鉴别金银花和山银花

【实验目的】

1. 了解 DNA 分子鉴别方法在中药鉴定中的应用。
2. 掌握金银花、山银花的位点特异性 PCR 鉴别方法。

【实验指导】

聚合酶链式反应（polymerase chain reaction，PCR）是一种模拟体内 DNA 复制过程的体外酶促合成特异性核酸片段的方法。通常需要两条位于待扩增片段两侧的寡聚核苷酸引物，这些引物分别与待扩增片段的正义链和反义链互补，使两引物之间的区域得以通过聚合酶链式反应扩增。扩增过程包括 DNA 变性、退火和延伸，如此重复多轮，DNA 片段以指数形式得以扩增。

DNA 分子鉴别通过比较物种间 DNA 分子的遗传差异来鉴别药材。DNA 分子具有遗传稳定性与化学稳定性，与性状鉴别、显微鉴别、理化鉴别方法相比，DNA 分子鉴别方法不受外界环境和药用植物发育阶段以及器官组织差异的影响，因而鉴别结果更为准确可靠。位点特异性 PCR 技术通过设计特异性引物，PCR 扩增和琼脂糖凝胶电泳可有效区分混伪药材。本实验设计特异性引物对金银花药材和山银花药材总 DNA 进行 PCR 扩增，对 PCR 产物进行凝胶电泳，根据凝胶电泳图谱可有效鉴别金银花与山银花。

【仪器与试剂】

1. 仪器

分析天平、研钵、微量移液枪、枪头、Eppendorf 管、高速冷冻离心机、水浴锅、凝胶成像仪等。

2. 试剂

CTAB 缓冲液、三氯甲烷、异戊醇、异丙醇、75% 乙醇、无菌水、Premix Taq 酶预混合 buffer、DNA marker、含 GelRed 核酸染料的 $10 \times$ loading buffer、$1 \times$ TAE 电泳缓冲液。

【实验材料】

1. 药材

金银花、山银花（灰毡毛忍冬花蕾）。

2. 引物

特异性引物 Lj－F：TTTATCCTTTTTTTGTTAGCGGTTGA，Lj－R：CTATCCCGACCATTCCC。按照要求，将引物稀释到工作浓度。

【实验内容与方法】

1. 金银花和山银花总 DNA 的提取

（1）将金银花和山银花的药材分别粉碎，并过 40 目筛。

（2）取约 20mg 粉末至 1.5ml 离心管中，加入 600μl 65℃预热的 CTAB 缓冲液，65℃水浴 30 分钟（每隔 10 分钟颠倒混匀）；

（3）12000r/min 离心 5 分钟；

（4）取 400μl 上清液，加入等体积的三氯甲烷 – 异戊醇（24:1），轻轻颠倒混匀 2 分钟；

（5）12000r/min 离心 5 分钟，取 300μl 上清液，加入等体积的三氯甲烷 – 异戊醇（24:1），轻轻颠倒混匀 2 分钟；

（6）12000r/min 离心 5 分钟；

（7）取 200μl 上清液，加入等体积 –20℃预冷的异丙醇，轻微混匀，至离心管内有白色絮状沉淀。若沉淀太少，可将离心管放入 –20℃冰箱冷冻 5 分钟左右；

（8）12000r/min 离心 5 分钟，小心弃上清，留下管内白色沉淀，加入 500μl 75% 乙醇重复漂洗两次。

（9）12000r/min 离心 3 分钟，小心弃掉漂洗液后，用白色 10μl 枪头吸出残留漂洗液；

（10）将离心管开盖放置于 40℃烘箱中约 20 分钟，待管内乙醇完全挥发后，加入 50μl 灭菌蒸馏水溶解提取的 DNA。

注意：1. 实验过程中所有离心管和枪头均需灭菌烘干后使用。2. 实验台面、打粉机均需认真清洁后使用。

2. 位点特异性 PCR 扩增

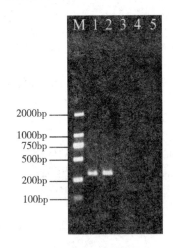

PCR 前将提取的 DNA 稀释，至模板浓度为 30 ~ 100ng/μl。选用 Premix Taq 酶预混合 buffer，配制 20μl 的 PCR 反应液：Premix Taq 酶预混合 buffer 10μl，10μmol · L^{-1}正反向引物（Lj – F、Lj – R）各 1μl，DNA 模板 1μl，灭菌水补充溶液体积至 20μl。

PCR 反应条件为：94℃ 5 分钟；34 个循环（94℃ 20 秒，51℃ 20 秒，72℃ 30 秒）；72℃ 3 分钟。

图 33 – 1　金银花和山银花药材 PCR 产物琼脂糖电泳图

Figure 33 – 1　The agarose gel electrophoresis of PCR products of Lonicerae Japonicae Flos and Lonicerae Flos

3. 琼脂糖凝胶电泳

在 20μl PCR 反应产物中加入 2.2μl 含 GelRed 核酸染料的 10 × loading buffer。混匀后，取 10μl 反应产物进行琼脂糖凝胶电泳，电泳时间约为 20 分钟，然后在凝胶成像仪中观察扩增结果（图 33 –1）。

【实验报告】

记录实验步骤与分析实验结果。

【思考题】

DNA 分子鉴别技术在生药鉴别中的适用范围？

Experiment 33　Molecular Identification of Lonicerae Japonicae Flos and Lonicerae Flos by Using Allele – specific PCR

【Objective】

1. To study the application of DNA molecular identification technology in identification of TCM.

2. To master the allele – specific PCR identification technique of Lonicerae Japonicae Flos and Lonicerae Flos.

【Principle】

Polymerase chain reaction (PCR) is a method of enzymatic synthesis specific nucleic acid fragments *in vitro*, which simulates the natural DNA replication process. PCR generally needs two oligonucleotide primers that flank the target region in duplex DNA. The primers are complementary to the fragments being extended. The primers are then extended on the template strand by DNA polymerase. After cycles of denaturation, annealing, and extension, DNA fragments were amplified exponentially.

DNA molecular identification could identify different medicinal materials by comparing the genetic diversity of different species. DNA molecules have genetic and chemical stability. Compared with character identification, microscopic identification and physical and chemical identification methods, DNA molecular identification is not affected by the external environment, the development stage of medicinal plants, and the differences of organs and tissues, and the identification results are more accurate and reliable. Allele – specific PCR technology can effectively distinguish pseudorandom herbs by designing specific primers, PCR amplification and agarose gel electrophoresis. In this experiment, specific primers were designed to amplify the PCR products from the total DNA of Lonicerae Japonicae Flos and Lonicerae Flos, which can effectively identify the adulteration of Lonicerae Japonicae Flos.

【Instruments and Reagents】

1. Instruments

Analytical balance, mortar, micropipette, pipette tips, eppendorf tube (1. 5ml), high speed freeze centrifuge, water bath, UV transilluminator.

2. Reagents

CTAB buffer, chloroform, isopentanol, isopropanol, 75% ethanol, ultrapure water, Premix Taq enzyme premix buffer, DNA Marker, 10 × loading buffer containing GelRed nucleic acid dye, 1 × TAE electrophoresis reagents.

【Materials】

1. Crude drugs

Lonicera japonica Flos and Lonicera Flos.

2. Primers

Lj – F: TTTATCCTTTTTTTGTTAGCGGTTGA, Lj – R: CTATCCCGACCATTCCC. According to the requirements of Genscript, dilute the primers to the working concentration.

【Experimental Procedures】

1. Extraction of total DNA of Lonicera japonica Flos and Lonicera Flos

（1）The crude drugs of Lonicera japonica Flos and Lonicera Flos were pulverized respectively, and screened through 40 – mesh sieve；

（2）Transfer 20mg powder into a 1.5ml Eppendorf tube and add 600μl CTAB solution, which was 65℃ preheated. The mixed solution was incubated for 30min at 65℃；

（3）Reverse Eppendorf tube gently every 10min；

（4）12000r/min centrifuge for 5min；

（5）Absorb 400μl supernatant, add equal volume of chloroform – isopentanol（24：1）, reverse gently several times for 2min；

（6）12000r/min centrifuge for 5min. Absorb 300μl supernatant and repeat the previous step；

（7）Absorb 200μl supernatant, add isopropanol precooled at −20℃ of equal volume and mix it well. White floccus precipitation can be seen in the centrifuge tube. If the precipitation is too small, the tube can be frozen in the refrigerator at −20℃ for about 5min；

（8）12000r/min centrifuge for 5min, discard the supernatant carefully；

（9）Add 500μl 75% ethanol and rinse twice, 12000r/min centrifuge for 3min, and discard the rinsing solution completely；

（10）Place the centrifuge tube in a 40℃ oven for about 20min. After the ethanol is completely dried, add 50μl distilled water to dissolve the extracted DNA.

Note: 1. All centrifuge tubes and pipette tips need to be sterilized and dried in the experiment. 2. The experimental table and powdering machines must be carefully cleaned before use.

2. Allele – specific PCR amplification

The DNA template needs to be diluted to a concentration of 30 ~ 100 ng/μl.

Choose the Premix Taq enzyme, and prepare the PCR reaction solution：

Premix mixed enzymeTaq	10μl
Primer Lj – F	1μl
Primer Lj – R	1μl

DNA template 　　　　　　　　　　　1μl

Ultrapure water 　　　　　　　　　　Add to 20μl

Put the reaction tube into the instrument of PCR, amplify according to the following procedure: 94℃ 5min, 34 cycle(94℃ 20 s, 51℃ 20 s, 72℃ 30 s), 72℃ 3min.

3. Agarose gel electrophoresis

Add 2. 2μl of 10 × loading buffer containing GelRed nucleic acid dye to 20μl of the reaction product. After mixing, 10μl of the reaction product was subjected to agarose gel electrophoresis, and the electrophoresis time was about 20min.

【Assignments】

Record the experimental procedure and analyze the results.

【Discussion】

What is the application scope of DNA molecular identification in the identification of crude drug?

实验三十四　天麻 HPLC 特征图谱鉴别

【实验目的】

掌握高效液相色谱特征图谱的建立方法。

【实验指导】

中药特征图谱是指中药材经过适当的处理后，采用一定的分析手段和仪器检测得到，能够标识其中各种组分群体特征的共有峰的图谱。它是一种综合的、可量化的鉴别手段，可用于鉴别中药材的真伪，评价中药材质量的均一性和稳定性。中药特征图谱可分为化学（成分）特征图谱和生物特征图谱。化学（成分）特征图谱多采用色谱、光谱技术测定，反映药材化学成分组成和种类上的特征。生物特征图谱则多采用分子标记技术测定，反映药材生物遗传学上的特征。比较来讲，HPLC 法具有高效、快速、灵敏、重现性好、应用范围广等特点，已成为中药色谱特征图谱研究的首选方法。建立药材 HPLC 特征图谱的一般程序包括：①样品收集；②供试品及对照品溶液的制备；③检测方法的确立，包括测定方法、供试品制备条件、测定条件的优化等；④方法学验证，包括精密度试验、重复性试验、稳定性试验等考察试验；⑤特征图谱建立，即根据多批次样品的 HPLC 图谱，建立共有模式，指定特征色谱峰。

【实验材料】

不同批次的天麻药材。

【仪器与试剂】

1. 仪器

分析天平、高效液相色谱仪、ODS - C_{18}反相色谱柱（4.6×250mm，5μm），超声波清洗器等。

2. 试剂

重蒸水、乙腈、磷酸、甲醇、对羟基苯甲醇、天麻素对照品、巴利森苷对照品、巴利森苷 B 对照品、巴利森苷 C 对照品、巴利森苷 E 对照品对照品等。

【实验内容与方法】

1. 样品溶液的制备

取本品粉末（过四号筛）约 0.5g，精密称定，置具塞锥形瓶中，精密加入 50% 甲醇 25ml，称定重量，超声处理（功率 500W，频率 40kHz）30 分钟，放冷，再称定重量，用 50% 甲醇溶液补足减失的重量，摇匀，滤过，取续滤液，即得。

2. 标准品溶液的制备

精密称取天麻素、对羟基苯甲醇、巴利森苷、巴利森苷 B、巴利森苷 C 及巴利森苷 E 对照品适量，置 10ml 量瓶中，加 50% 甲醇溶解并稀释至刻度，摇匀，制成浓度分别为

0. 30、0. 10、0. 60、0. 30、0. 10、0. 40mg/ml 的混合对照品溶液。

3. 色谱条件

色谱柱：ODS - C$_{18}$反相色谱柱（4. 6×250mm，5μm）；流动相：乙腈（A）- 0. 1%磷酸（B），梯度洗脱，洗脱程序见表 34 - 1；检测波长 220nm；流速 0. 8ml/min；柱温 30℃；进样体积 3μl。

表 34 - 1　梯度洗脱程序

时间（min）	A（%）	B（%）
0 ~ 10	3→10	97→90
10 ~ 15	10→12	90→88
15 ~ 25	12→18	88→82
25 ~ 35	18→18	82→82
35 ~ 37	18→95	82→5

4. HPLC 特征图谱的建立

（1）平衡高效液相色谱仪至基线平稳，精密吸取 3μl 供试品溶液注入液相色谱仪，按上述色谱条件进行色谱分析，数据采集时间为 40 分钟，得到供试品溶液的 HPLC 图谱。

（2）精密吸取 3μl 对照品溶液注入液相色谱仪，按上述色谱条件进行色谱分析，数据采集时间为 40 分钟，得到对照品的 HPLC 图谱。

（3）共有峰的确定。收集 10 组样品测试数据。以天麻素峰为参照峰，以其保留时间为基准，计算其余各峰的相对保留时间（R_{RT}）（式 34 - 1）。相对保留时间的相对偏差小于3%，可确定为共有峰。

$$R_{RT(i)} = \frac{RT_{(i)}}{RT_{(s)}} \tag{34 - 1}$$

式中，$RT_{(i)}$为各色谱峰的保留时间，$RT_{(s)}$为参照峰的保留时间。

（4）记录各色谱峰的保留时间，采用国家药典委员会颁布的《中药色谱指纹图谱相似度评价系统》（2012 版），对 10 批样品的图谱及数据进行综合评价，生成天麻对照特征图谱（图 34 - 1）。

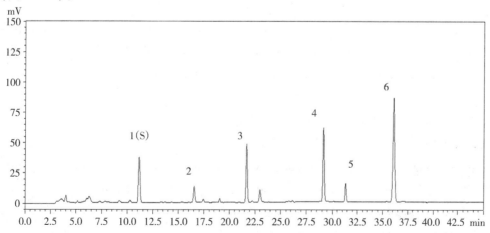

图 34 - 1　天麻对照特征图谱

Figure 34 - 1　HPLC characteristic chromatogram of Gastrodiae Rhizoma

1. 天麻素（gastrodin（S））；2. 对羟基苯甲醇（p - hydroxybenzyl alcohol）；3. 巴利森苷 E（barrison E）；

4. 巴利森苷 B（barrison B）；5. 巴利森苷 C（barrison C）；6. 巴利森苷（barrison glycosides）

【实验报告】

1. 记录本组测试得到的天麻 HPLC 特征图谱。
2. 标记天麻特征图谱中共有峰并计算相对保留时间。

【思考题】

1. HPLC 特征图谱中参照峰应该如何选择?
2. 阐述中药特征图谱的优缺点。

Experiment 34　Identification of Gastrodiae Rhizoma by HPLC Characteristic Chromatogram

【Objective】

1. To master the establishment method of HPLC characteristic chromatogram.

【Principle】

The characteristic chromatogram of TCM refers to the chromatogram that can identify the common peaks of various constituents and groups after proper treatment of TCM by means of certain analytical methods and instruments. It is a comprehensive and quantifiable identification method, which can be used to identify the authenticity of Chinese medicinal materials and evaluate the quality uniformity and stability of Chinese medicinal materials. The characteristic chromatogram of TCM can be divided into chemical characteristic chromatogram and biological characteristic chromatogram. Chemical characteristic chromatogram is mostly determined by chromatographic and spectral techniques, reflecting the characters of the chemical composition and types of the medicinal materials. Biological characteristic chromatogram is mostly determined by molecular marker technology, reflecting the biogenetic characters of medicinal materials. Comparatively, HPLC is characterized by high efficiency, high speed, sensitivity, good reproducibility and wide application range, etc. , and has become the first choice for the study of TCM characteristic chromatogram. The general procedures for establishing HPLC characteristic chromatogram of crude drugs include: ①Sample collection. ②Preparation of test and reference solutions. ③The establishment of the detection method, including the determination method, the preparation condition of the test, the optimization of the determination condition, etc. ④Method validation, including precision test, repeatability test, stability test and other investigation tests. ⑤The establishment of the characteristic chromatogram, according to the HPLC chromatograms of multiple batches of samples, generate a common model, identify the characteristic peaks.

【Materials】

Gastrodiae Rhizoma from different habitats.

【Instruments and Reagents】

1. Instruments

HPLC, ODS – C₁₈ reversed phase chromatograph column (4.6 × 250mm, 5μm), analytic balance, ultrasonic cleaner.

2. Reagents

Redistilled water, acetonitrile(HPLCgrade), phosphoric acid, methanol, gastrodin CRS, parishin CRS, parishin B CRS, parishin C CRS, parishin E CRS.

【Experimental Procedures】

1. Preparation of test solution

Weigh accurately 0.5g of the powder(through No.4 sieve) to a stoppered conical flask, add accurately 25ml of 50% methanol and weight, ultrasonicate for 30min, allow to cool, weight again, replenish the loss of the solvent with 50% methanol and mix well, filter the supernatant and use the successive filtrate as test solution.

2. Preparation of reference solution

Dissolve separately a quantity of gastrodin CRS, parishin CRS, parishin B CRS, parishin C CRS, parishin E CRS, accurately weighed, in 50% methanol to produce a solution containing 0.30, 0.10, 0.60, 0.30, 0.10, 0.40mg in 1ml.

3. Chromatographic system

Column: ODS – C₁₈ reversed phase chromatograph column (4.6 × 250mm, 5μm); Mobile phase: acetonitrile as the mobile phase A and 0.1% solution of phosphoric acid as the mobile phase B, the gradient elution program is shown in Table 34 – 1. The spectrophotometer is set at 220nm. The flow rate is 0.8ml/min. The column temperature is 30℃. The injection volume is 3μl.

Table 34 – 1 The gradient elution program

Time(min)	Mobile Phase A(percent, V/V)	Mobile Phase B(percent, V/V)
0 – 10	3→10	97→90
10 – 15	10→12	90→88
15 – 25	12→18	88→82
25 – 35	18→18	82→82
35 – 37	18→95	82→5

4. Establishment of HPLC characteristic spectrum

(1) Counterpoise the HPLC by flowing mobile phase until the baseline is stable. Inject accurately 3μl of test solution, measure according to the above chromatographic system with running time of the chromatogram 40min, and get the HPLC chromatograph of Gastrodiae Rhizoma.

(2) Inject accurately 3μl of reference solution, measure according to the above chromatographic system with running time of the chromatogram 40min, and get the HPLC chromatograph of reference solution.

(3) Collect the test date of the total 10 groups. Choose the peak of Gastrodin as the reference,

calculate the relative retention time of the other peaks (R_{RT}) (Formula 34 − 1). If the RSD of relative retention time is less than 3%, it was regarded as the common peak.

$$R_{RT(i)} = \frac{RT_{(i)}}{RT_{(s)}} \qquad (34-1)$$

Comments: $RT_{(i)}$ is the retention time of the main peaks, $RT_{(s)}$ is the retention time of reference peak.

(4) Using Similarity evaluation system for chromatographic fingerprint of TCM (2012 edition) issued by the National Pharmacopoeia Committee to evaluate the chromatogram and data of 10 batches of samples comprehensively, and generate a control characteristic chromatogram.

【Assignments】

1. Record the HPLC characteristic chromatogram of Gastrodiae Rhizoma.

2. Record the relative retention time of all common peaks in the HPLC characteristic chromatogram.

【Discussion】

1. How to select the reference peak in HPLC characteristic chromatogram?

2. State the advantages and disadvantages of HPLC characteristic chromatogram of TCM.

实验三十五　银杏叶 HPLC 特征图谱鉴别

【实验目的】

1. 了解中药指纹图谱/特征图谱。
2. 掌握中药指纹图谱/特征图谱技术在质量控制中的应用。

【实验指导】

中药含有的化学成分种类繁多并且复杂，很难完全表征所有化合物，单一的指标成分也难以反映其质量的优劣。中药指纹图谱技术具有整体性和模糊性的特点，是实现鉴别中药真实性及评价质量一致性的可行模式，已广泛应用于中药材及中药制剂的质量控制。其中以色谱法最为常用，尤其是高效液相色谱法。建立银杏叶 HPLC 指纹图谱能够比较全面地反映其所含成分，用于银杏叶的鉴别和全面的质量控制。

银杏叶为银杏科植物银杏 *Ginkgo biloba* L. 的干燥叶，研究表明，银杏叶的主要成分为黄酮类和萜类内酯类成分。黄酮类化合物在植物体内常与糖结合，主要以槲皮素、山奈酚和异鼠李素的单糖苷、二糖苷、三糖苷的形式存在，糖基的连接位点主要是 3 位羟基，如芦丁、异鼠李素 – 3 – *O* – 葡萄糖苷等，另外还含有双黄酮类，包括银杏双黄酮、7 – 去甲基银杏双黄酮、异银杏双黄酮等；萜类内酯是银杏叶的特征性成分，主要包括二萜内酯（银杏内酯 A、B、C、M 等）、倍半萜内酯（白果内酯）；此外，银杏叶还含有很多其他类型的活性成分，如有机酸类、原花青素类、儿茶素类等。

【仪器与试剂】

1. 仪器

高效液相色谱仪、超声波清洗器、Agilent ZORBAX Eclipse Plus C_{18} 柱（100mm × 2.1mm，1.8μm）、移液管、容量瓶、具塞锥形瓶等。

2. 试剂

甲醇、乙腈（色谱纯）、甲酸（色谱纯）、二甲基亚砜（DMSO）、芦丁对照品、7 – 去甲基银杏双黄酮对照品等。

【实验材料】

银杏叶粉末（过四号筛）。

【实验步骤】

1. 溶液的制备

（1）供试品溶液的制备取银杏叶粉末（过四号筛）约 0.5g，精密称定，置具塞锥形瓶中，精密加入甲醇 10ml，超声处理 30 分钟（500W，40kHz），取出放冷，过滤，取续滤液，滤纸放入原锥形瓶中，残渣精密加 75% 甲醇 10ml，超声 30 分钟，放冷，过滤，合并两次

149

滤液，摇匀，用 0.22μm 的滤膜过滤，取续滤液，即得。

（2）参照物溶液的制备取芦丁对照品适量，精密称定，加甲醇溶解；取 7 - 去甲基银杏双黄酮对照品适量，精密称定，先用 DMSO 溶解再用甲醇稀释；分别制成每 1ml 含 0.1mg 的参照物溶液。

2. 色谱条件

色谱柱为 Agilent ZORBAX Eclipse Plus C$_{18}$ 柱（100mm × 2.1mm，1.8μm）；流动相为 0.05% 甲酸水（A）和乙腈 - 甲醇（8：2，V/V）（B），梯度洗脱，洗脱程序见表 35 - 1；检测波长 360nm；流速 0.3ml/min；柱温 40℃；进样体积 2μl。银杏叶药材 HPLC 特征图谱如图 35 - 1 所示。

表 35 - 1　梯度洗脱程序

时间（分钟）	流动相 A（%）	流动相 B（%）
0 ~ 18	85	15
18 ~ 19	85→84	15→16
19 ~ 33	84	16
33 ~ 34	84→80	16→20
34 ~ 45	80	20
45 ~ 53	80→74	20→26
53 ~ 65	74	26
65 ~ 66	74→58	26→42
66 ~ 80	58	42
80 ~ 81	58→50	42→50
81 ~ 90	50	50
90 ~ 100	50→10	50→90
100 ~ 105	10	90

3. 特征峰标定及相对保留时间的测定

根据对照特征图谱，对供试品图谱（图 35 - 1）中的特征峰进行指认，其中 2 个峰应分别与芦丁及 7 - 去甲基银杏双黄酮参照物峰保留时间相同，分别记为峰 S$_1$ 和峰 S$_2$。以 S$_1$ 计算特征峰 1 ~ 7 的相对保留时间，以 S$_2$ 计算特征峰 8 ~ 11 的相对保留时间，其相对保留时间应在规定值的 ±10% 之内。规定值为：1.00（峰 1）、1.79（峰 2）、1.90（峰 3）、2.38（峰 4）、4.40（峰 5）、5.54（峰 6）、0.95（峰 7）、1.00（峰 8）、1.15（峰 9）、1.17（峰 10）及 1.28（峰 11）。

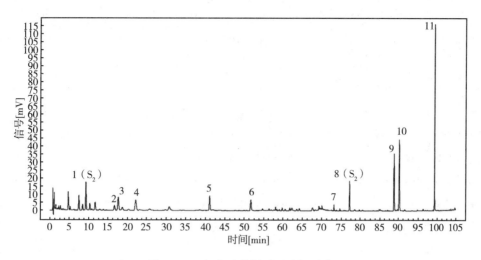

图 35 - 1　银杏叶药材对照特征图谱

Figure 35 - 1　The reference fingerprint of Ginkgo Folium

1. 芦丁 rutin（S1）；

2. 槲皮素 - 3 - O - 葡萄糖基（1 - 2）鼠李糖苷（quercetin - 3 - O - D - glucosyl - (1 - 2) - L - rhamnoside）；

3. 山柰酚 - 3 - O - 芸香糖苷（kaempferol - 3 - O - rutinoside）；4. 水仙苷（isorhamnetin - 3 - O - rutinoside）；

5. 3 - O - {2 - O[- 6 - O - （对羟基 - 反 - 香豆酰）- 葡萄糖基]- 鼠李糖基}- 槲皮素

（quercetin - 3 - O - 2" - (6" - p - coumaroyl) - glucosyl - rhamnoside）；

6. 3 - O - {2 - O[- 6 - O - （对羟基 - 反 - 香豆酰）- 葡萄糖基]- 鼠李糖基}- 山柰酚

（kaempferol - 3 - O - 2" - (6" - p - coumaroyl) - glucosyl - rhamnoside）；

7. 穗花杉双黄酮（amentoflavone）；8. 7 - 去甲基银杏双黄酮（bilobetin）（S2）；

9. 银杏双黄酮（ginkgetin）；10. 异银杏双黄酮（isoginkgetin）；11. 金松双黄酮（sciadopitysin）

【实验报告】

1. 记录银杏叶 HPLC 特征图谱的实验内容及结果。

2. 根据与银杏叶药材对照图谱的比对及特征峰的指认结果，对银杏叶药材的真伪作出鉴别。

【思考题】

1. HPLC 特征图谱的优缺点有哪些?

2. 目前为止，《中国药典》《欧洲药典》及《美国药典》现行版对银杏叶中总黄酮苷的含量测定都是采用酸水解法间接测定苷元，请查阅文献，分析采用此方法测定的原因及此方法有何不足之处。

Experiment 35　Identification of Ginkgo Folium by HPLC Characteristic Fingerprint Chromatography

【Objective】

1. To understand the principle of HPLC characteristic fingerprint chromatography.

2. To master the application of the characteristic fingerprint chromatography technology in crude drugs.

【Principle】

Traditional Chinese medicine contains a wide variety and complex chemical components, which is difficult to fully characterize all compounds, and a single index component is difficult to reflect its quality. Chromatographic fingerprint has been gradually recognized as an effective and holistic approach to identify the authenticity and evaluate the consistency of quality. Chromatography is the most commonly used, especially HPLC. The establishment of HPLC fingerprint can comprehensive analysis of Ginkgo Folium.

Ginkgo Folium is a dry leaf of *Ginkgo biloba* L. The research has demonstrated that the components of Ginkgo Folium are flavonoids and terpene trilactones. In plants, flavonoids often links glycosyl, mainly in the form of monoglycosides, diglycosides and trisglycosides of quercetin, kaempferol and isorhamnetin. The linkage sites of glycosyl groups are mainly 3 – hydroxy groups, such as rutin, isorhamnetin – 3 – O – glucoside. Moreover, it also contains biflavonoids, including ginkgetin, bilobetin, isoginkgetin, etc. Terpene trilactones are characteristic components of leaf including diterpenoids lactone(ginkgolide A, B, C, M) and sesquiterpene lactone(bilobalide). In addition, Ginkgo Folium. also contain many other types of active ingredients, such as organic acids, proanthocyanidins and catechins.

【Instruments and Reagents】

1. Instruments

HPLC apparatus, Agilent ZORBAX Eclipse Plus C_{18} column (100mm × 2.1mm, 1.8μm), ultrasonic cleaner, pipette, volumetric flask, conical flask.

2. Reagents

Methanol, acetonitrile(HPLC grade), formic acid(HPLC grade), dimethyl sulfoxide(DMSO), rutin CRS and bilobetin CRS.

【Materials】

Ginkgo Folium.

【Experimental Procedures】

1. Preparation of solutions

(1)Test solution: Each sample powder(0.5g, through No.4 Sieve) was accurately weighed and extracted ultrasonically(500W, 40kHz) with 10ml of MeOH in a 50ml conical flask for 30min. The extracted solution was filtered until cooling to room temperature. The residue was re – extracted with 10ml of 75% MeOH. The combined extracts were filtered through 0.22μm filter membrane and stored at 4℃ before HPLC analysis.

(2)Reference solution: Rutin was weighed and dissolved in MeOH, and bilobetin was prepared with DMSO firstly. Then, reference solution was prepared by diluting with methanol to make a solution containing 0.10mg per 1ml.

2. Chromatographic condition

Column: Agilent ZORBAX Eclipse Plus C_{18} column (100mm × 2.1mm, 1.8μm); mobile phase: 0.05% formic acid in H_2O(phase A) and a mixture of ACN and MeOH(8:2, *V/V*)(phase B), elute in a gradient program as Table 35 − 1; wavelength: 360nm; low rate: 0.3ml/min; column temperature: 40℃; injection volume: 2μl.

3. Assay

Determination of characteristic peaks and calculation their relative retention times. 11 characteristic peaks should be present in the chromatogram, of which two peaks should have the same retention time as the peaks of rutin and bilobetin, respectively, are recorded as peak S_1 and peak S_2, respectively. S_1 was used to calculate the relative retention time of characteristic peaks 1 − 7, and S_2 was used to calculate the relative retention time of characteristic peaks 8 − 11. The relative retention time should be within the specified value plus or minus 10% : 1.00(peak 1), 1.79(peak 2), 1.90(peak 3), 2.38(peak 4), 4.40(peak 5), 5.54(peak 6), 0.95(peak 7), 1.00(peak 8), 1.15(peak 9), 1.17(peak 10) and 1.28(peak 11).

Table 35 − 1　The gradient elution program

Time(min)	Phase A(%)	Phase B(%)
0 − 18	85	15
18 − 19	85→84	15→16
19 − 33	84	16
33 − 34	84→80	16→20
34 − 45	80	20
45 − 53	80→74	20→26
53 − 65	74	26
65 − 66	74→58	26→42
66 − 80	58	42
80 − 81	58→50	42→50
81 − 90	50	50
90 − 100	50→10	50→90

【Assignments】

1. Record the experimental procedures and results.

2. Refer to the characteristic HPLC chromatograms of Ginkgo Folium and the results of calculated relative retention times of characteristic peaks, please authenticating the samples of "Ginkgo Folium".

【Discussion】

1. What are the advantages and disadvantages of the characteristic HPLC chromatograms in

quality control of TCMs.

2. In current pharmacopoeia including Ch. P. , United States Pharmacopoeia (USP) , and European Pharmacopoeia(EP) ,the normal method for the quantitative analysis of flavonol glycosides were determined indirectly with acidic hydrolysis followed by determination of the resulting aglycones. Please refer to the literature and analyze the reasons and the deficiencies of this method.

实验三十六 一标多测法同时测定黄芩中 四种黄酮类成分

【实验目的】

1. 了解一标多测法的原理。
2. 掌握一标多测法在生药多成分测定中的应用。

【实验指导】

1. 一标多测法

生药有效成分多为一类或几类同系物组成。一标多测法（quantitative analysis of multi – constituents by single – marker，QAMS）是在测定中药多指标成分时，依据在一定范围内（线性范围）成分的量（质量或浓度）与检测器响应成正比的原理，引入相对校正因子的概念，以样品中某一典型成分（价廉、易得、有活性）为参照物，建立该成分与其他待测成分之间的相对校正因子，通过相对校正因子计算其他成分含量的一种方法。用公式表示如下：

$$f_{si} = \frac{f_s}{f_i} = \frac{A_S/C_S}{A_i/C_i} \tag{36-1}$$

式中，f_{si} 为参照物 s 对待测成分 i 的校正因子，A_S 为参照物 s 的峰面积或峰高，C_S 为参照物 s 的浓度，A_i 为某待测成分 i 的峰面积或峰高，C_i 为某待测成分 i 的浓度。

2. 相对校正因子的测定方法

相对校正因子常采用以下两种方法测定：

（1）斜率法 取系列不同浓度参照物及待测成分的对照品，配制参照物及待测成分的对照品溶液，注入高效液相色谱仪或气相色谱仪，用最小二乘法以质量或浓度对峰面积进行线性回归（应代入原点），按公式（36-2）计算相对校正因子。

$$f_{sx} = \frac{f_s}{f_x} = \frac{1}{k_{sx}} = \frac{k_s}{k_x} \tag{36-2}$$

式中，f_{sx} 为参照物 s 与待测成分 x 的相对校正因子，k_x 为某待测成分 x 的标准曲线斜率，k_s 为参照物 s 的标准曲线斜率。

（2）多点法 配制不同浓度的混合对照品溶液，以多个浓度点计算所得校正因子的平均值作为相对校正因子，其计算公式如式（36-3）所示：

$$f_{k/s} = \frac{C_s \times A_k}{C_k \times A_s} \tag{36-3}$$

式中，$f_{k/s}$ 为相对校正因子；C_s 为参照物浓度；A_s 为参照物峰面积；C_k 为其他对照组分浓度；A_k 为其他对照组分峰面积。

【仪器与试剂】

1. 仪器

高效液相色谱仪、超声波清洗器、Agilent Zorbax Extend – C18 柱（250mm × 4.6mm，5μm）、容量瓶、具塞锥形瓶等。

2. 试剂

甲醇、乙腈（色谱纯）、磷酸、乙醇、黄芩苷对照品、汉黄芩苷对照品、黄芩素对照品、汉黄芩素对照品等。

【实验材料】

黄芩粉末（过四号筛）。

【实验步骤】

以黄芩苷为参照物，测定汉黄芩苷、黄芩素和汉黄芩素的相对校正因子和相对保留时间，用一标多测法测定黄芩药材中汉黄芩苷、汉黄芩素、黄芩素的含量。

1. 溶液的制备

（1）供试品溶液的制备　取黄芩粉末（过四号筛）约 0.1g，精密称定，置具塞锥形瓶中，精密加入 70% 甲醇 50ml，密塞，称定重量，超声处理 15 分钟，放冷，再称定重量。用 70% 甲醇补足减失的重量，摇匀。滤过，取续滤液，作为供试品溶液。

（2）对照品溶液的制备　分别取黄芩苷、汉黄芩苷、汉黄芩素、黄芩素对照品 10mg，精密称定，置 10ml 量瓶中，用甲醇溶解并稀释至刻度，作为对照品储备溶液。吸取对照品储备液，稀释制备成适宜浓度的对照品工作溶液。

2. 色谱条件

色谱柱为 Agilent Zorbax Extend – C$_{18}$ 柱（250mm×4.6mm，5μm）；流动相为 0.1% 磷酸（A）和乙腈（B），梯度洗脱，洗脱程序见表 36 – 1；检测波长 276nm；流速 1.0ml/min；柱温 30℃；进样体积 10μl。黄芩药材 HPLC 图谱如图 36 – 1 所示。

表 36 – 1　梯度洗脱程序

时间（分钟）	流动相 A（%）	流动相 B（%）
0 ~ 10	78→75	22→25
10 ~ 15	75	25
15 ~ 25	75→68	25→32
25 ~ 30	68→60	32→40
30 ~ 35	60	40
35 ~ 40	60→50	40→50
40 ~ 45	50→5	50→95
45 ~ 50	5	95
50 ~ 53	5→78	95→22
53 ~ 60	78	22

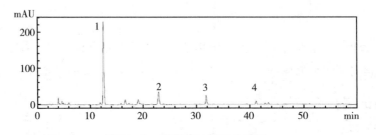

图 36 – 1　黄芩药材 HPLC 图谱

Figure 36 – 1　HPLC chromatogram of ScutellariaeRadix

1. 黄芩苷（baicalin）；2. 汉黄芩苷（wogonoside）；3. 黄芩素（waicalein）；4. 汉黄芩素（wogonin）

3. 相对校正因子及相对保留时间的测定

以黄芩苷为参照物，采用斜率法测定汉黄芩苷、汉黄芩素、黄芩素的相对校正因子。

计算待测物峰与参照物峰保留时间的比值，即得相对保留时间。相对保留时间 = 待测物峰保留时间/参照峰保留时间。

4. 含量测定

分别精密吸取对照品溶液与供试品溶液，注入液相色谱仪，测定。以黄芩苷对照品为参照，根据相对保留时间（允许范围为 ±5%），确定待测成分汉黄芩苷、汉黄芩素、黄芩素的色谱峰。按外标法计算黄芩苷的含量，按照公式（36 – 1）分别计算汉黄芩苷、汉黄芩素、黄芩素的含量。

【实验报告】

1. 记录一标多测法的实验内容及结果。

2. 以黄芩苷为参照物，测定汉黄芩苷、汉黄芩素、黄芩素的相对校正因子及相对保留时间；计算黄芩药材中黄芩苷、汉黄芩苷、黄芩素和汉黄芩素的含量。

【思考题】

1. 阐述一测多评方法的适用范围。

2. 一测多评法的优缺点有哪些?

Experiment 36　Simultaneous Quantification Four Flavonoids in Scutellariae Radix Using Quantitative Analysis of Multi – constituents by Single Marker

【Objective】

1. To understand the principle of the method "quantitative analysis of multi – constituents by single – marker".

2. To learn to the application of the method "quantitative analysis of multi – constituents by single – marker" in crude drugs.

【Principle】

The effective constituents in a crude drug are often structural homologues. The method "quantitative analysis of multi – constituents by single – marker" (QAMS) is proposed to overcome the shortage of reference substances when multi – constituent quantification is carried out. The principle of the method is that within a certain linear range, the amount of analyte (mass or concentration) is directly proportional to the detector response. To do this, the concept of relative correction factor is introduced. Firstly, a representative constituent in crude drug is chosen as reference substance, due to its cheap cost and easy availability. Then, the relationship between reference substance and other constituents to be tested is correlated via relative correction factor.

Finally, other constituents can be quantified by employing the relative correction factor. The principle can be elucidated by the following formula.

$$f_{si} = \frac{f_s}{f_i} = \frac{A_S/C_S}{A_i/C_i} \qquad (36-1)$$

where f_{si} is the relative correction factor of reference substance s to the test constituent i, A_S is the peak area or peak height of reference substance s, C_S is the concentration of reference substance s, A_i is the peak area or peak height of the test constituent i, and C_i is the concentration of the test constituent i.

2. Determination of relative correction factor

The following two strategies can be used to determine relative correction factor.

（1）Slope method: Prepare the working solutions of reference substance and constituents to be quantified at a series of concentrations, inject the the working solutions into the system of HPLC or GC, construct the linear regression formulas by plotting the peak area versus the concentration with least square linear regression (the coordinate origin should be introduced). The relative correction factor is thus calculated according to the following formula.

$$f_{sx} = \frac{f_s}{f_x} = \frac{1}{k_{sx}} = \frac{k_s}{k_x} \qquad (36-2)$$

where f_{sx} is the correction factor of reference substance relative to test constituent x, k_s is the slope of reference substance curve, and k_x is the slope of test constituent curve.

（2）Multi – point method: Prepare the working solutions of reference substance and test constituents at a series of concentrations, calculate the relative correction factors at each concentration according to the following formula, average the obtained values as the relative correction factor.

$$f_{k/s} = \frac{C_s \times A_k}{C_k \times A_s} \qquad (36-3)$$

where $f_{k/s}$ is the correction factor relative of reference substance s relative to test constituent x, C_s is the concentration of reference substance, A_s is the peak area of reference substance, C_k is the concentration of test constituent, and A_k is the peak area of test constituent.

【Instruments and Reagents】

1. Instruments

HPL Capparatus, Agilent Zorbax Extend – C18 column (250mm × 4.6mm, 5μm), ultrasonic cleaner, volumetric flask, conical flask.

2. Reagents

Methanol, acetonitrile (HPLC grade), phosphoric acid, ethanol, baicalin CRS, wogonoside CRS, wogonin CRS, baicalein CRS.

【Materials】

Scutellariae Radix.

【Experimental Procedures】

Calculate the relative correction factors and relative retention times of wogonoside, wogonin and baicalein, using baicalin as reference substance. Calculate the contents of wogonoside, wogonin and baicalein in Scutellariae Radix, using QAMS method.

1. Preparation of solutions

（1）Test solution：Weigh accurately 0. 1g of the powder of Scutellariae Radix（through No. 4 sieve）to a stopper conical flask, accurately add 50ml of 70% methanol and weigh. Ultrasonicate for 15min, cool and weigh again. Replenish the loss of weight with 70% methanol. Mix well and filter, and use the successive filtrate as the test solution.

（2）Reference solution：Weigh accurately 10mg of baicalin CRS, wogonoside CRS, wogonin CRS and baicalein CRS to a 10ml volumetric flask, dissolve in methanol and dilute to the volume, use as stocking solution. Dilute the stocking solution with methanol to produce working solutions at a series of concentrations.

2. Chromatographic condition

Column：Agilent Zorbax Extend – C18 column（250mm × 4. 6mm, 5μm）; mobile phase: 0. 1% phosphoric acid（phase A）and acetonitrile（phase B）, elute in gradient as Table 36 – 1; wavelength：276nm; flow rate：1. 0ml/min; column temperature：30℃; injection volume：10μl.

Table 36 – 1　The gradient elution program

Time（min）	Phase A（%）	Phase B（%）
0 – 10	78→75	22→25
10 – 15	75	25
15 – 25	75→68	25→32
25 – 30	68→60	32→40
30 – 35	60	40
35 – 40	60→50	40→50
40 – 45	50→5	50→95
45 – 50	5	95
50 – 53	5→78	95→22
53 – 60	78	22

3. Determination of relative correction factor and relative retention time

Calculate the correction factors of wogonoside, wogonin and baicalein relative to baicalin, using the slope method. Calculate relative retention times of wogonoside, wogonin and baicalein, using baicalin as reference substance. Relative retention time = Retention time of baicalin/Retention time of test constituent.

4. Assay

Inject accurately a quantity of reference working solution and test solution, respectively, into the column. Using baicalin as reference substance, identify the chromatographic peaks corresponding to the test constituents of wogonoside, wogonin and baicalein, with the aid of relative retention times (tolerance range is ±5%). Calculate the content of baicalin by using external reference method, calculate the contents of wogonoside, wogonin and baicalein by using QAMS method.

【Assignments】

1. Record the experimental procedures and results.

2. Calculate the relative correction factors and relative retention times of wogonoside, wogonin and baicalein, using baicalin as reference substance. Calculate the contents of baicalin, wogonoside, wogonin and baicalein in Scutellariae Radix.

【Discussion】

1. What is the applicable scope of QAMS?
2. What are the advantages and disadvantages of QAMS?

实验三十七 生药质量标准研究与制订

【实验目的】

1. 熟悉生药质量标准研究与制订的程序。
2. 掌握生药质量标准的主要内容。

【实验指导】

1. 生药质量标准研究与制订程序

主要包括拟定研究方案、准备样品及标准物质、开展实验研究、起草质量标准草案、编写起草说明、标准复核与终审等步骤。其流程图如图37-1所示。

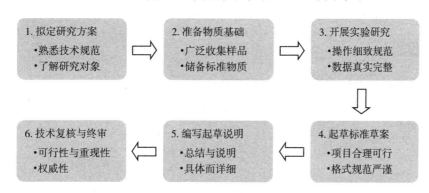

图 37-1　生药质量标准研究与制订程序流程图

Figure 37-1　Process flow chart of study and formulation of crude drug quality standard

2. 生药质量标准的主要内容

生药质量标准的主要内容一般包括：名称、来源、性状、鉴别、检查、特征图谱、浸出物、含量测定等项。各项目的具体要求如下：

（1）名称包括中文名、汉语拼音及拉丁名。

（2）来源包括原植（动）物的科名、中文名、拉丁名及药用部位、采收季节、产地加工方法等。

（3）性状主要指对该药材的形状、大小、表面（色泽、特征）、质地、断面、气、味等特征进行感官描述，如用眼看（较细小的可借助于放大镜或解剖镜）、手摸、鼻闻、口尝等。应抓住主要特征描述，文字简练，用语准确。鉴别多植（动）物来源的药材，其性状无明显区别者，可合并描述；有明显区别者，应分别描述。无论是根、根茎、藤茎、果实、皮类药材，应尽量多描述断面特征，以便对破碎药材或饮片进行鉴别。相关技术规范可参考《中国药典》四部0212药材和饮片检定通则。

（4）鉴别用经验鉴别、显微鉴别、理化鉴别和DNA分子标记鉴别对该药材进行真伪鉴别。相关技术规范可参考《中国药典》四部2001显微鉴别法、0301一般鉴别试验、0400光谱法、0500色谱法等通则。

（5）检查对该药材的杂质、水分、灰分、有害或有毒物质等进行的限量检查或含量测

161

定，并制订限度。相关技术规范可参考《中国药典》四部 2301 杂质检查法、0832 水分测定法、2302 灰分测定法、2321 铅、镉、铜、汞、砷测定法、2341 农药残留量测定法、2331 二氧化硫残留量测定法、2351 黄曲霉毒素测定法等通则。

（6）特征图谱中药特征图谱是从中药指纹图谱中选取若干专属性强的色谱峰或色谱峰组合形成特征指纹图谱，用于该药材的专属性鉴别。

（7）浸出物结合用药习惯、药材质地及已知的化学成分类别等选定适宜的溶剂，测定该药材浸出物含量以控制质量。相关技术规范可参考《中国药典》四部 2201 浸出物测定法。

（8）含量测定用化学、物理或生物的方法，对该药材含有的有效成分、指标成分或类别成分进行测定，以评价其内在质量的项目和方法。含量测定的内容包括：测定成分的选择、含量测定方法的选择、含量测定方法的验证、含量限度的制订等。

【实验步骤】

选择某一生药，查阅相关文献资料，拟定质量标准制订或修订方案，开展相应实验研究，根据研究结果起草质量标准草案，并编写起草说明。

【实验报告】

起草该生药的质量标准草案，并编写起草说明。

【思考题】

所起草的质量标准草案中，每个项目在控制该生药质量时起到何种作用？

Experiment 37　Establishement of Quality Standard for Crude Drug

【Objective】

1. To know the establishment procedures of quality standard for crude drugs.
2. To master the method of establishing a quality standard.

【Principle】

1. Establishment procedures of quality standard

The following six steps are essential to establishing a quality standard, viz. ① proposing a research protocol; ② preparing samples and reference substances; ③ conducting experiments; ④ drafting quality standard; ⑤ compiling elucidation materials; ⑥ technical checking and final evaluation.

2. Main contents of the quality standard of a crude drug

The quality standard of a crude drug consists of the following items, viz. name, origin, description, identification, test, characteristic chromatogram, extractive, and assay. The specific requirements of each item are as follows:

（1）Name：This item contains Chinese name and its phonetic symbols，as well as the Latin name of the crude drug.

（2）Origin：This item contains family，Chinese name and Latin name of the botanical or animal origin，as well as the medicinal part，harvesting time and the process method in the producing area.

（3）Description：This item is to describe the shape，size，external，texture，fracture，odour and taste acquired by human senses. The description should be focused on the main characters in a concise and accurate style. For those multi – original crude drugs，if there are no obvious differences among species，the identification characters can be described together，if there are visible differences among species，the identification characters should be described separately. Fraction characters should be paid more attention so as to identify the broken crude drug or decoction pieces. Relevant technical requirements can refer to General Chapter 0212 in Volume Ⅳ of Chinese Pharmacopoeia.

（4）Identification：This item is to identify the authenticity of the crude drug by using the methods of empirical identification，microscopical identification，DNA molecular marker identification and physicochemical identification. Relevant technical requirements can refer to General Chapters 2001，0301，0400，and 0500 in Volume Ⅳ of Chinese Pharmacopoeia.

（5）Test：This item is to determine the limits of foreign matter，water，ash，and hazardous substances in the crude drug. Relevant technical requirements can refer to General Chapters 2301，0832，2302，2321，2341，2331 and 2351 in Volume Ⅳ of Chinese Pharmacopoeia.

（6）Characteristic chromatograms：This item is to establish characteristic fingerprint by selection of distinctive chromatographic peaks from a chromatographam，for the specific identification of crude drug.

（7）Extractive：This item is to determine the extractive of crude drug extracted by suitable solvent according to the texture and the type of chemical constituents. Relevant technical requirements can refer to General Chapter 2201 in Volume Ⅳ of Chinese Pharmacopoeia.

（8）Assay：This item is to determine the effective constituents，marker constituents，or category constituents in crude drug by chemical，physical or biological methods. The details includes：the choice of analyte and determination method，the validation of determination method，and the establishment of content limit.

【Experimental procedures】

For a given crude drug，propose the research protocol based on extensive iterature retrieval，then conduct the experiments accordingly，draft the quality standard on the basis of obtained results，and compile the elucidation materials.

【Assignments】

Draft the quality standard for the given crude drug and compile the elucidation materials.

【Discussion】

What is the role of each item in the drafted quality standard for controlling the quality of crude drug?

163

附录　生药鉴定专业词汇

斑点	spot
半复粒淀粉粒	half compound starch granule
胞间隙	intercellular space
胞间腺毛	interspace glandular hair
胞腔	cell lumen
薄壁细胞	parenchymatous cells
薄壁组织	parenchyma
薄层扫描仪	thin layer scanner
薄层色谱法	thin – layer chromatography
饱和的	saturated
比移植	R_f value
边缘效应	edge effect
表面观	surface view
表面特征	surface character
表皮	epidermis
不定根	adventitious
不规则的	irregular
不明显的	inconspicuous
不平坦的	uneven
草酸钙簇晶	clusters of calcium oxalate
层纹	annular striation
车轮纹	wheel radial striations
沉淀	precipitation
橙皮苷结晶	hesperidin crystal
初生构造	primary structure
初生木质部	primary xylem
初生皮层	primary cortex
除去杂质	removal of foreign matter
穿孔	perforation
垂周壁	anticlinal wall
醇溶性浸出物	ethanol – soluble extractives

次生构造	secondary structure
次生木质部	secondary xylem
粗糙的	coarse
簇晶	cluster crystal
萃取	extraction
大小	size
淡	weak
导管	vessel
等度洗脱	isocratic elution
滴定液	volumetric solution
点样	application of sample
点状维管束	spotted vascular bundles
电泳法	electrophoresis methods
淀粉粒	starch granule
定量分析	quantitative analysis
定量限	limit of quantitation
定性分析	qualitative analysis
动态平衡	a dynamic equilibrium
段、节	segment
断面	fracture
对照品溶液	reference solution
对照药材	referencecrude drug
盾状毛	peltate hair
反相液相色谱法	reversed phase liquid chromatography
方法学验证	method validation
方晶	prism
芳香的	aromatic
纺锤形	fusiform
非腺毛	nonglandular hair
分光光度法	spectrophotometry
分光光度计	spectrophotometer
分离度	resolution
分泌道	secretory canals

分泌物	secretion
分泌组织	secretory tissue
分配色谱法	partition chromatography
粉性的	starchy
丰富的	abundant
峰高	peak height
峰宽	peak width
峰面积	peak area
复粒淀粉粒	compound starch granule
副卫细胞	subsidiary cell
干燥失重	loss on drying
高效液相色谱法	high performance liquid chromatography
高效预制板	pre – coated HPTLC plate
铬	cadmium
根	root
根被	velamen
根迹维管束	root trace bundle
根茎	rhizome
汞	mercury
供试品溶液	test solution
固定相	stationary phase
固相萃取	solid phase extraction
管胞	tracheid
管状中柱	siphonostele
光辉带	light line
硅胶	silica gel
果皮	pericarp
果实	fruit
过载	overloading
海绵组织	spongy tissue
含水量	moisture content
痕	scar

横切面	transverse section
烘干法	oven drying method
后生皮层	metaderm
厚壁组织	sclerenchyma
厚角组织	collenchyma
糊粉粒	aleurone grain
花	flower
环纹	annulations
环形的	annular
灰分	ash
灰分测定	determination of ash
挥发油测定	determination of volatile oil
回收率	recovery
茴香醛溶液	anisaldehyde solution
火试	fire – based test
基线	base line
基线漂移	baseline drift
基线噪声	baseline noise
甲酸	formic acid
坚实的	compact
坚硬的	hard
间断的	interrupted
检测限	limit of detection
检识	detection
角质层	cuticle
角质样的	horny
结晶囊	crystal sac
解离组织	disintegrated tissue
近，类	sub –
近方形	subquadrate
近三角形	subtriangular
浸出物测定	determination of extractives

浸渍	macerate
晶纤维	crystal fiber
精密度	precision
菊花心	radial striations
具缘纹孔	bordered pit
聚集的	grouped
菌丝	hypha
凯氏带	Casparian strip
凯氏点	Casparian dots
颗粒状	granular
孔沟	pit canal
块、瓣、部分	section
宽的	broad
类多角形	subpolygonal
类圆形	subrounded
冷浸提法	cold maceration method
离子交换色谱法	ion exchange chromatography
理化鉴定	physical and chemical identification
理论塔板数	theoretical plate
连续展开	continuous development
连珠状	beaded
晾干	dried in the air
裂缝	crack/cleft
菱形	rhombic
流动相	mobile phase
流速	flow rate
螺纹的	spiral
落皮层	rhytidome
氯仿	chloroform
脉岛数	vein islet number
醚溶性浸出物	ether – soluble extractives
密集的	dense

明显的	distinct
木	wood
木薄壁细胞	xylem parenchyma
木化的	lignified
木间韧皮部	interxylary phloem
木射线	xylem ray
木栓	cork/phellem
木栓层	cork
木栓石细胞	corksclereid
木栓素	suberin
木栓细胞	cork cell
木纤维	wood fiber
木质部	xylem
目镜显微量尺	ocular micrometer
内标法	internalcalibration
内果皮	endocarp
内涵韧皮部	included phloem
内皮层	endodermis
黏液细胞	mucilage cell
凝胶色谱法	gel chromatography
农药残留	pesticide residue
胚乳	endosperm
皮	bark
皮层	cortex
皮孔	lenticel
平周壁	periclinal wall
脐点	hilum
脐点	hilum
气	odour/odor
气孔	stoma
气孔数	stomatal number
气孔指数	stomatal index

铅	lead
全草	herb
热浸提法	hot extraction method
韧皮部	phloem
韧皮射线	phloem ray
韧型纤维	libriform fiber
乳汁管	laticiferous tube
三生构造	tertiary structure
散在的	scattered
色谱峰保留时间	retention time of peak
色素细胞	pigment cell
色泽	color
砂晶	sandy crystal
筛板	sieve plate
筛管	sieve tube
筛管群	sieve tube group
筛域	sieve area
晒干	dried in the sun
上表皮	upper epidermis
上行展开	ascending development
射线	ray
砷	arsenic
石细胞	sclereid
示差折光检测器	refractive index detector
束中形成层	fascicular cambium
树脂道	resin canal
栓内层	phelloderm
双韧管状中柱	amphiphloic siphonostele
双韧维管束	bicollateral vascular bundle
双向展开	two dimensional development
水分测定	determination of water
水合氯醛溶液	chloral hydrate solution

水溶性浸出物	water – soluble extractives
水试	water – based test
死时间	dead time
死体积	dead volume
松脆的	lax and fragile
酸不溶性灰分	acid – insoluble ash
髓	pith
羧甲基纤维素钠	sodium carboxymethylcellulose
特征色谱峰	characteristic peak
特征图谱	characteristic chromatogram
梯度洗脱	gradient elution
梯度展开	gradient development
梯纹的	scalariform
甜的	sweet
条斑	bands
铜	copper
透光率	transmittance
突起	protrusions
拖尾系数	the extent of tailing
拖尾因子	tailing factor
脱气	degas
脱盐	desalting
外标法	external calibration
外表	externally
外果皮	exocarp
外胚乳	perisperm
外皮层	exodermis
外韧维管束	collateral vascular bundle
网纹的	reticulated
网纹细胞	reticulated cell
网眼，网状组织	reticulations
网状中柱	dictyostele

微	slightly
微量升华	microsublimation
维管束	vascular bundle
味	taste
纹孔	pit
纹理	striation
无限外韧维管束	unclosed collateral bundle
吸附剂	adsorbent
吸附色谱法	adsorption chromatography
吸光度	absorbance
稀疏的	sparse
洗净泥土	washed clean
系统适用性	system suitability
下表皮	lower epidermis
下行展开	descending development
下皮	hypodermis
下皮纤维	hypodermal fiber
纤维	fiber
纤维管胞	fiber tracheid
纤维束	fiber bundles
显色剂	chromogenic reagent
显微化学反应	microchemical reaction
显微鉴定	microscopical identification
显微特征	microscopical characters
线性	linearity
腺鳞	glandular scale
腺毛	glandular hair
相对，较	relatively
相对标准偏差	relative standard deviation
镶嵌细胞层	parquetry layer
辛辣的	pungent
信噪比	signal – to – noise ratio

星点	star spots
星状毛	stellate hair
形成层	cambium
形状	shape/form
性状鉴定	macroscopical identification
须根	fibrous root/rootlet
续滤液	successive filtrate
盐酸	hydrochloric acid
支持细胞	supporting cell
叶	leaf
叶绿体	chloroplast
叶脉	vein
液-液萃取	liquid - liquid partitioning
乙醚	ether
异常构造	anomalous structure
异型维管束	abnormal vascular bundles
易弯曲的	flexible
易折断的	easily broken
阴干	dried in the shade
饮片	decoction pieces
荧光	fluorescence
荧光淬灭	quench the fluorescence
荧光分析法	fluorimetric analysis
荧光检测器	fluorescence detector
荧光指示剂	fluorescent indicator
油管	vittae/oil duct
油室	oil cavity
油细胞	oil cell
有限外韧维管束	closed collateral bundle
预制板	pre - coated TLC plate
原点	origin
原动物鉴定	identification of original animal

原生中柱	protostele
原植物鉴定	identification of original plant
圆柱形	cylindrical
圆锥形	conical
云锦状花纹	cloudy – brocaded patterns
杂质	foreign matter
杂质检查	determination of foreign matter
载玻片	microslide
载台显微量尺	stage micrometer
栅表细胞比	palisade ratio
栅栏组织	palisadetissue
窄的	narrow
粘性的	viscous
展开	development
展开缸	developing tank
展开剂前沿	solvent front
展开溶剂	development agent
展开系统	development system
折断面	fracture
针晶	raphide
蒸馏	distillation
正相液相色谱法	normal phase liquid chromatography
支根	branch root
纸色谱法	paper chromatography
指纹图谱	fingerprint
指示液	indicator solution
质地	texture
中果皮	mesocarp
中空的	hollow
中药	Chinese medicines
中药材	Chinese medicinal material
中柱	stele

中柱鞘	pericycle
钟乳体	cystolith
种子	seed
重金属及有害物质	heavy metals and harmful elements
重现性	reproducibility
周木维管束	amphivasal vascular bundle
周皮	periderm
周韧维管束	amphicribral vascular bundle
皱纹	wrinkle
朱砂点	spot of oil cavity
主根	main root
柱晶	styloid
柱色谱	column chromatography
专属性	specificity
准确度	accuracy
子叶细胞	cotyledon cell
紫外光灯	ultraviolet light
紫外可见光检测器	ultraviolet visible detector
总灰分	total ash
总浸出物	total extractives
纵切面	longitudinal section
组织构造	histological structure

彩图

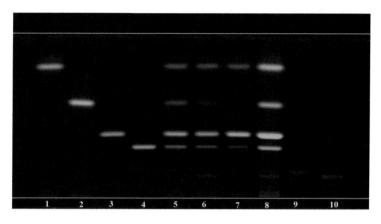

图 6 – 1 黄连薄层色谱图

Figure 6 – 1 Thin layer chromatography of Coptidis Rhizome

1. 黄连碱（coptisine hydrochloride CRS）；2. 表小檗碱（epiberberine hydrochloride CRS）；3. 小檗碱（berberine hydrochloride CRS）；

4. 巴马汀（palmatine hydrochloride CRS）；5. 味连（Rhizome of *Coptidis chinensis*）；6. 雅连（Rhizome of *Coptidis deltoidea*）；

7. 云连（Rhizome of *Coptidis teeta*）；8. 黄连对照药材（Coptidis Rhizome reference crude drug）

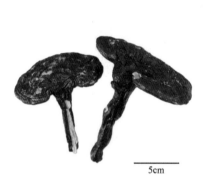

5cm

图 11 – 1 灵芝（赤芝）性状图

Figure 11 – 1 Macroscopic characteristics of Ganoderma（fruiting body of *G. lucidum*）

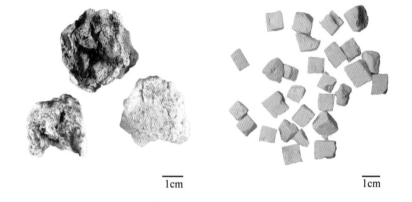

1cm   1cm

图 11 – 2 茯苓性状图

Figure 11 – 2 Macroscopic characteristics of Poria

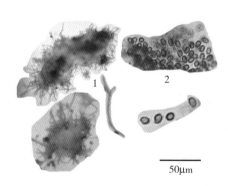

50μm

图 11 – 3 灵芝粉末显微特征图

Figure 11 – 3 Powder characteristics of Ganoderma（fruiting body of *G. lucidum*）

1. 菌丝（hyphae）；2. 孢子（spores）

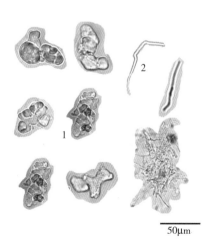

50μm

图 11 – 4 茯苓粉末显微特征图

Figure 11 – 4 Powder characteristics of Poria

1. 菌丝团（hypha ball）；2. 菌丝（hyphae）

1

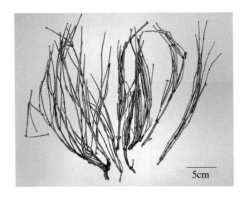

图 12 - 1　麻黄（草麻黄）性状图

Figure 12 - 1　Macroscopic characteristics of Ephedrae Herba（stem of *E. sinica*）

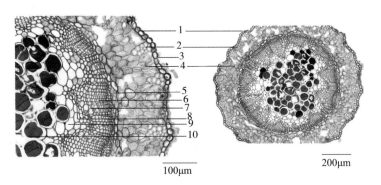

图 12 - 2　草麻黄（茎节间）横切面

Figure 12 - 2　Transverse section of Ephedrae Herba（stem of *E. sinica*）

1. 表皮细胞（epidermis cells）；2. 下皮纤维（hypodermal fibres）；3. 气孔（stomata）；
4. 皮层（cortex）；5. 中柱鞘纤维（pericyclic fibre bundles）；6. 韧皮部（phloem）；
7. 形成层（cambium）；8. 木质部（xylem）；
9. 环髓纤维（perimedullary fibres）；10. 髓（pith）

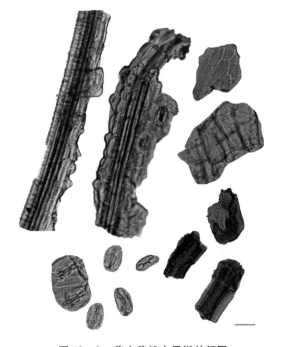

图 12 - 3　草麻黄粉末显微特征图

Figure 12 - 3　Powder characteristics of Ephedrae Herba（stem of *E. sinica*）

1. 表皮细胞（epidermis cells）；2. 气孔（stoma）；
3. 嵌晶纤维（sandy crystals）；4. 棕色块（brown lumps）

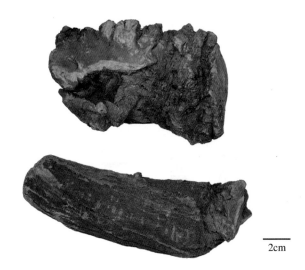

图 13 - 1　大黄性状图

Figure 13 - 1　Macroscopic characteristics of Rhei Radix et Rhizoma（root and rhizome of *R. palmatum*）

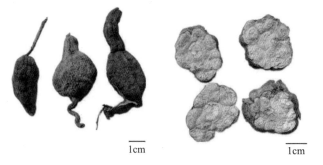

图 13 - 2　何首乌性状图

Figure 13 - 2　Macroscopic characteristics of Polygoni Multiflori Radix

2

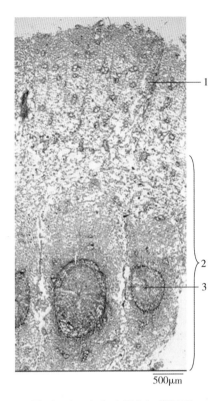

图 13 – 3 大黄（根茎）横切面

Figure 13 – 3 Transverse section of Rhei Radix et Rhizoma（rhizome of *R. palmatum*）

1. 韧皮部（phloem）；2. 髓（pith）；
3. 异型维管束（abnormal vascular bundles）

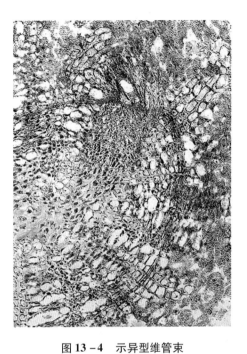

图 13 – 4 示异型维管束

Figure 13 – 4 Showing abnormal vascular bundles

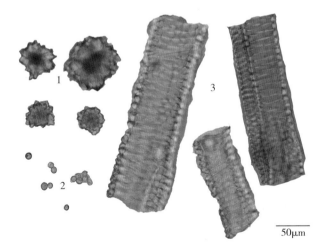

图 13 – 5 大黄粉末显微特征图

Figure 13 – 5 Powder characteristics of Rhei Radix et Rhizoma

1. 草酸钙簇晶（clusters of calcium oxalate）；2. 淀粉粒（starch granules）；3. 导管（vessels）

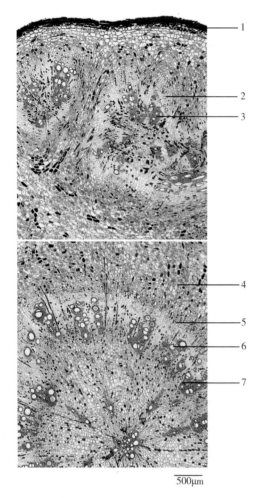

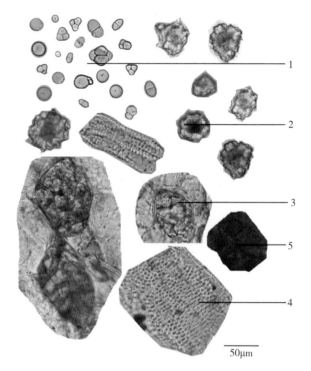

图 13 - 6　何首乌（块根）横切面

**Figure 13 - 6　Tansverse section of
Polygoni Multiflori Radix**

1. 木栓层（cork）；

2. 异型维管韧皮部（phloem in abnormal vascular bundles）；

3. 异型维管束木质部（xylem in abnormal vascular bundles）；

4. 韧皮部（phloem）；5. 形成层（cambium）；

6. 木质部（xylem）；7. 木纤维（xylem fibre）

图 13 - 7　何首乌粉末显微特征图

**Figure 13 - 7　Powder characteristics of
Polygoni Multiflori Radix**

1. 淀粉粒（starch granules）；

2. 草酸钙簇晶（clusters of calcium oxalate）；

3. 棕色细胞（brown cells）；4. 导管（vessels）；

5. 棕色块（brown masses）

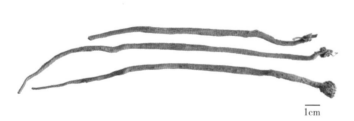

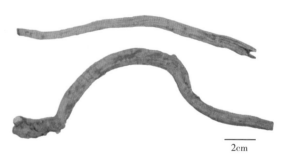

图 14 - 1　牛膝性状图

**Figure 14 - 1　Macroscopic characteristics of
Achyranthis Bidentatae Radix**

图 14 - 2　川牛膝性状图

**Figure 14 - 2　Macroscopic characteristics of
Cyathulae Radix**

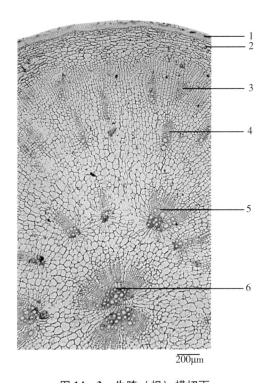

图 14 - 3　牛膝（根）横切面

Figure 14 - 3　Tansverse section of Achyranthis Bidentatae Radix

1. 木栓层（cork）；2. 栓内层（phelloderm）；

3. 外轮维管束（outermost whorl vascular bundle）；

4. 第二轮维管束（second whorl vascular bundle）；

5. 第三轮维管束（third whorl vascular bundle）；

6. 中心维管束（central vascular bundle）

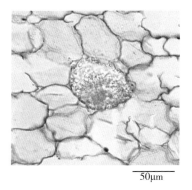

图 14 - 4　示草酸钙砂晶

Figure 14 - 4　Showing sand crystals of calcium oxalate

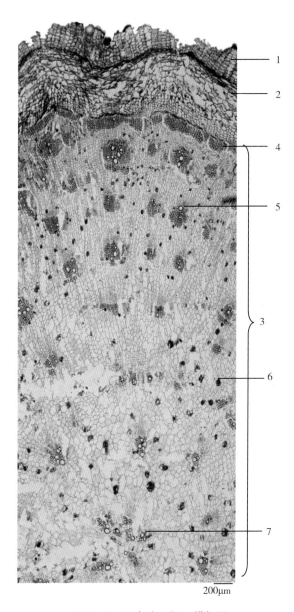

图 14 - 5　川牛膝（根）横切面

Figure 14 - 5 Tansverse section of Cyathulae Radix

1. 木栓层（cork）；2. 栓内层（phelloderm）；

3. 中柱（vascular cylinder）；4. 木纤维（xylary fibres）；

5. 三生维管束（tertiary vascular bundles）；

6. 草酸钙结晶（crystals of calcium oxalate）；

7. 中央次生维管束（secondary vascular bundles at centre）

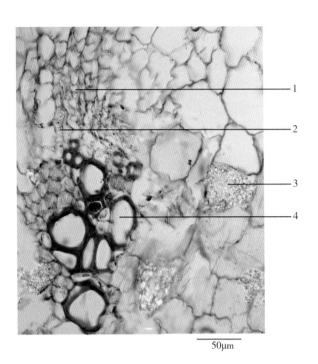

图 14－6　三生维管束放大图

Figure 14－6　Tertiary vascular bundles magnified

1. 韧皮部（phloem）；2. 形成层（cambium）；

3. 草酸钙砂晶（sand crystals of calcium oxalate）；

4. 木质部（xylem）

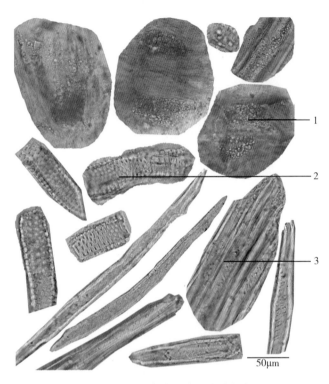

图 14－7　川牛膝粉末显微特征图

Figure 14－7　Powder characteristics of Cyathulae Radix

1. 草酸钙砂晶（sand crystals of calcium oxalate）；

2. 具缘纹孔导管（bordered pitted vessels）；

3. 纤维（fibres）

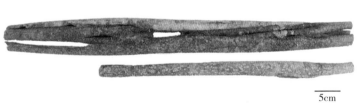

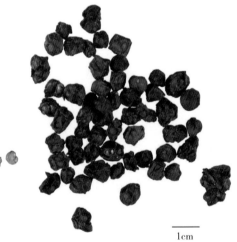

图 15－1　厚朴性状图

**Figure 15－1　Macroscopic characteristics
of Magnoliae Officinalis Cortex**

图 15－2　五味子性状图

**Figure 15－2　Macroscopic characteristics
of Schisandrae Fructus**

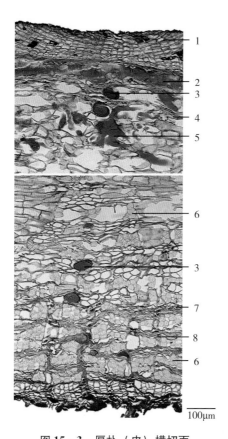

图 15 - 3　厚朴（皮）横切面

Figure 15 - 3　Transverse section of Magnoliae Officinalis Cortex

1. 木栓层（cork）；2. 石细胞环带（ring of sclereid）；
3. 油细胞（oil cells）；4. 皮层（cortex）；
5. 石细胞群（groups of sclereid）；6. 纤维束（fibre bundles）；
7. 韧皮部（phloem）；8. 韧皮射线（phloem rays）

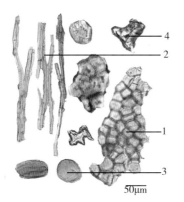

图 15 - 4　厚朴粉末显微特征图

Figure 15 - 4　Main powder characteristics of Magnoliae Officinalis Cortex（*M. officinalis*）

1. 木栓细胞（cork cells）；2. 纤维（fibres）；
3. 油细胞（oil cells）；4. 石细胞（sclereid）

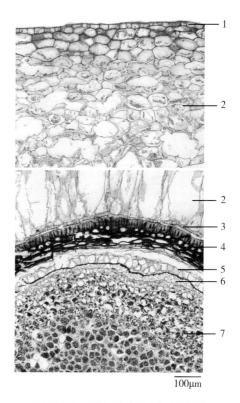

图 15 - 5　五味子（果实）横切面

Figure 15 - 5　Transverse section of Schisandrae Fructus

1. 外果皮（exocarp）；2. 中果皮（mesocarp）；
3. 内果皮（endocarp）；4. 种皮（testa）；
5. 油细胞层（oil cell layer）；6. 种皮内表皮
（inner epidermal cells of testa）；7. 胚乳（endosperm）

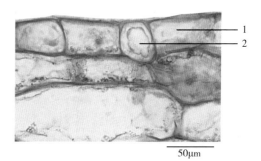

图 15 - 6　外果皮放大

Figure 15 - 6　Exocarp magnified

1. 外果皮（exocarp）；2. 油细胞（oil cell）

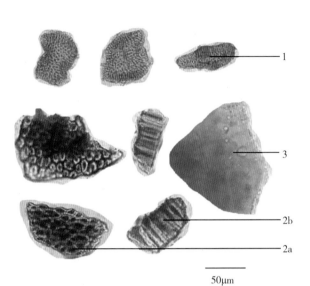

图 15 - 7　五味子果实粉末显微特征图

Figure 15 - 7　Main powder characteristics of Schisandrae Fructus

1. 种皮内层石细胞（inner layer sclereid of testa）；

2. 种皮表皮石细胞（epidermal sclereid）

〔a. 表面观（surface view）; b. 侧面观（lateral view）〕；

3. 果皮表皮细胞（epidermal cells of pericarp）

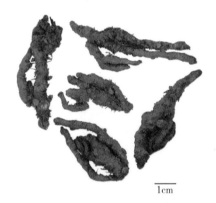

图 16 - 1　黄连（味连）性状图

Figure 16 - 1　Macroscopic characteristics of Coptidis Rhizoma（rhizome of *C. chinensis*）

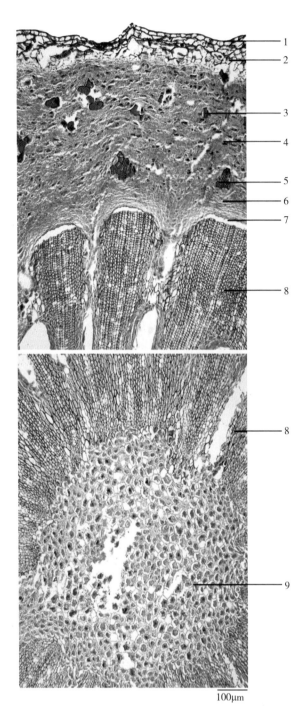

图 16 - 2　味连（根茎）横切面

Figure 16 - 2　Transverse section of Coptidis Rhizoma（rhizome of *C. chinensis*）

1. 表皮（epidermis）; 2. 木栓层（cork）; 3. 石细胞群（sclereid）;

4. 皮层（cortex）; 5. 中柱鞘纤维束（pericyclic fibre bundles）;

6. 韧皮部（phloem）; 7. 形成层（cambium）;

8. 木质部（xylem）; 9. 髓（pith）

8

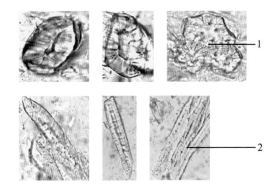

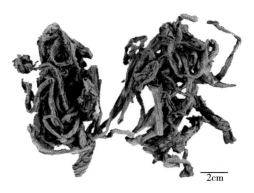

图16-3 黄连粉末显微特征图

Figure 16-3 Powder characteristics of Coptidis Rhizoma

1. 石细胞（sclereid）；2. 纤维（fibres）

图17-1 大青叶性状图

Figure 17-1 Macroscopic characteristics of Isatidis Folium

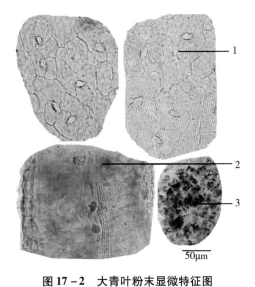

图17-2 大青叶粉末显微特征图

Figure 17-2 Main powder characteristics of Isatidis Folium

1. 叶下表皮细胞（lower epidermal cells of leaf）；

2. 叶断面观，示叶肉组织（section view of leaf, showing mesophyll tissue）；

3. 叶肉细胞含蓝色颗粒状物（mesophyll cells containing numerous blue pigment granules）

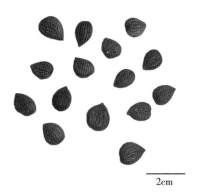

图18-1 苦杏仁性状图

Figure 18-1 Macroscopic characteristics of Armeniacae Semen Amarum

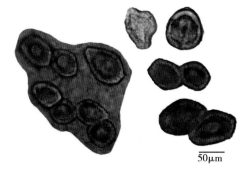

图18-2 苦杏仁粉末显微特征图

Figure 18-2 Main powder characteristics of Armeniacae Semen Amarum

1. 石细胞（sclereid）

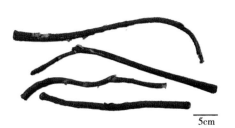

图19-1 甘草性状图

Figure 19-1 Macroscopic characteristics of lycyrrhizae Radix et Rhizoma（root of *G. uralensis*）

9

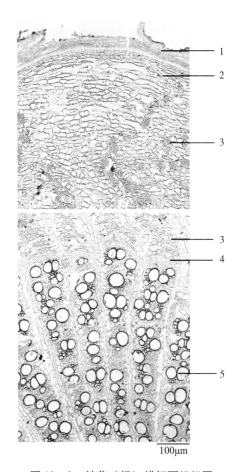

图 19 – 2　甘草（根）横切面组织图

Figure 19 – 2　Tansverse section of Glycyrrhizae

Radix et Rhi – zoma（root of *G. uralensis*）

1. 木栓层（cork）；2. 皮层（cortex）；3. 韧皮部（phloem）；

4. 形成层（cambium）；5. 木质部（xylem）；导管（vessels）

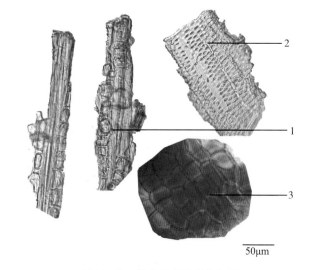

图 19 – 3　甘草粉末显微特征图

Figure 19 – 3　Main powder characteristics of Glycyrrhizae

Radix et Rhizoma（*G. uralensis*）

1. 纤维（fibers）；2. 导管（vessels）；3. 木栓细胞（cork cells）

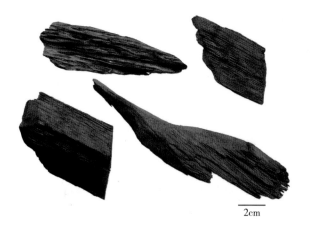

图 20 – 1　沉香（白木香）性状图

Figure 20 – 1　Macroscopic characteristics of

Aquilariae Lignum Resinatum

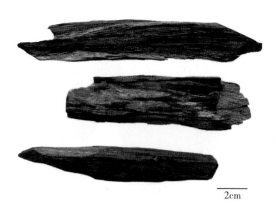

图 20 – 2　沉香（进口）性状图

Figure 20 – 2　Macroscopic characteristics of

imported Aquilariae

10

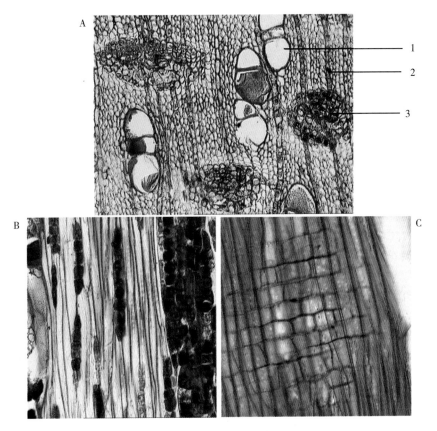

图 20 – 3　沉香组织三切面

Figure 20 – 3　Three section of Aquilariae Lignum Resinatum

A. 横切面（tansverse section）；B. 径向纵切面（radial longitudinal section）；

C. 切向纵切面（tangential longitudinal section）

1. 导管（vessels）；2. 射线（rays）；3. 木间韧皮部（interxylary phloem）

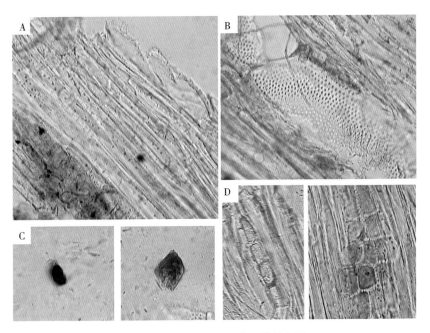

图 20 – 4　国产沉香粉末显微特征图

Figure 20 – 4　Main powder characteristics of Aquilariae Lignum Resinatum

A. 纤维管胞（tracheid fibers）；B. 导管（vessels）；C. 树脂团块（resin piece）；D. 射线（rays）

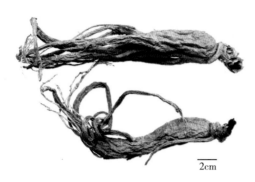

图 21 – 1　人参性状图

Figure 21 – 1　Macroscopic characteristics of Ginseng Radix et Rhizoma

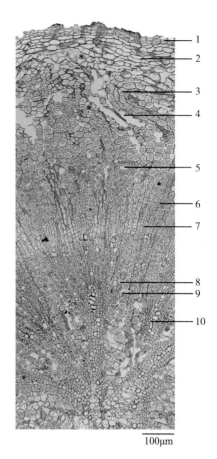

图 21 – 3　人参（根）横切面

Figure 21 – 3　Transverse section of Ginseng Radix et Rhizoma（root）

1. 木栓层（cork）；2. 栓内层（phelloderm）；3. 韧皮射线（phloem ray）；
4. 裂隙（cleft）；5. 树脂道（resin canals）；6. 韧皮部（phloem）；
7. 形成层（cambium）；8. 木射线（xylem ray）；
9. 草酸钙簇晶（clusters of calcium oxalate）；10. 木质部（xylem）

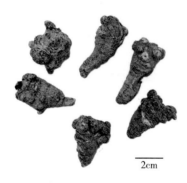

图 21 – 2　三七性状图

Figure 21 – 2　Macroscopic characteristics of Notoginseng Radix et Rhizoma

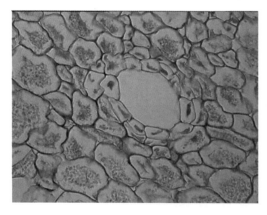

图 21 – 4　示树脂道

Figure 21 – 4　Showing resin canals

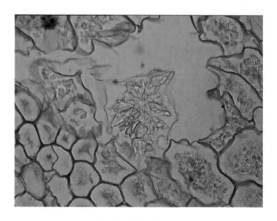

图 21 – 5　示草酸钙簇晶

Figure 21 – 5　Showing clusters of calcium oxalate

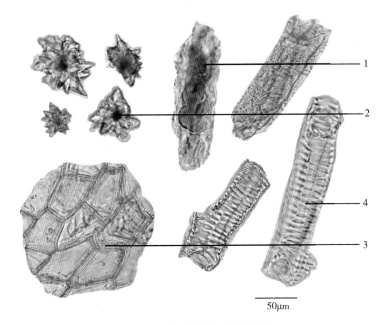

图 21 –6　人参粉末显微特征图

Figure 21 –6　Main powder characteristics of Ginseng Radix et Rhizoma

1. 树脂道碎片（fragments of resin canals）；2. 草酸钙簇晶（clusters of calcium oxalate）；

3. 木栓细胞（cork cells）；4. 导管（vessels）

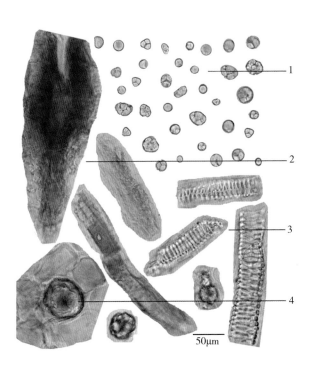

图 21 –7　三七根粉末显微特征图

Figure 21 –7　Main powder characteristics of
Notoginseng Radix et Rhizoma

1. 淀粉粒（starch granules）；2. 树脂道（resin canals）；

3. 导管（vessels）；4. 草酸钙簇晶（clusters of calcium oxalate）

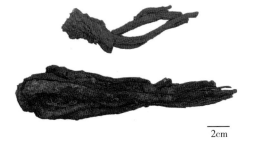

图 22 –1　当归性状图

Figure 22 –1　Macroscopic characteristics of
Angelicae Sinensis Radix

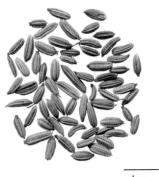

图 22 –2　小茴香性状图

Figure 22 –2　Macroscopic characteristics of
Foeniculif Fructus

13

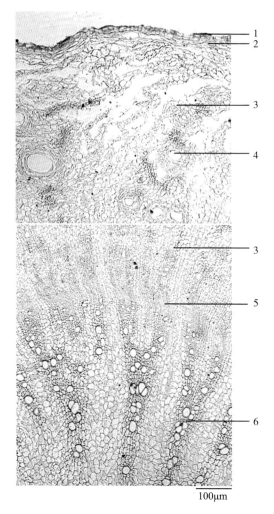

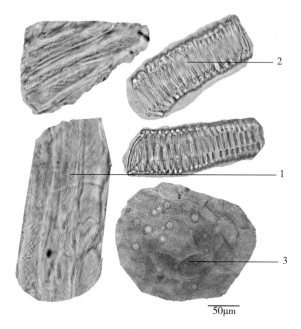

图 22 -5　当归粉末显微特征图

Figure 22 -5　Main powder characteristics of Angelicae Sinensis Radix

1. 韧皮薄壁细胞（phloem parenchymatous cells）；

2. 导管（vessels）；3. 油室碎片（fragments of oil cavities）

图 22 -3　当归（根）横切面

Figure 22 -3　Transverse section of Angelicae Sinensis Radix

1. 木栓层（cork）；2. 皮层（cortex）；

3. 韧皮部（phloem）；4. 油室（oil cavities）；

5. 形成层（cambium）；6. 木质部（xylem）

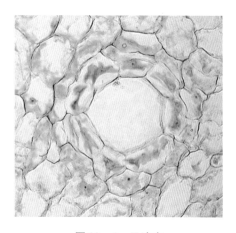

图 22 -4　示油室

Figure 22 -4　Showing oil cavities

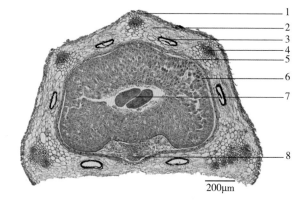

图 22 -6　小茴香（果实）横切面

Figure 22 -6　Transverse section of Foeniculif Fructus

1. 外果皮（exocarp）；2. 中果皮（mesocarp）；3. 油管（vittae）；

4. 维管束（vascular bundles）；5. 内果皮（endocarp）；

6. 胚乳（endosperm）；7. 胚（embryo）；

8. 种脊维管束（rhaphe vascular bundles）

14

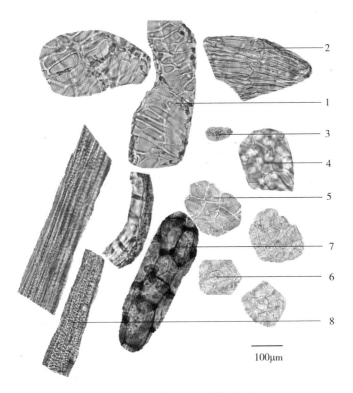

图 22 - 7　小茴香粉末显微特征图

Figure 22 - 7　Main powder characteristics of Foeniculif Fructus

1. 网状细胞（reticulated cells）；2. 内果皮镶嵌细胞（interdigitating cells）；

3. 草酸钙簇晶（clusters of calcium oxalate）；4. 胚乳细胞（endosperm cells）；

5. 外果皮表皮细胞（exocarp epidermal cells）；6. 气孔（stomata）；

7. 油管碎片（vittae debris）；8. 木薄壁组织细胞（xylem parenchyma cells）

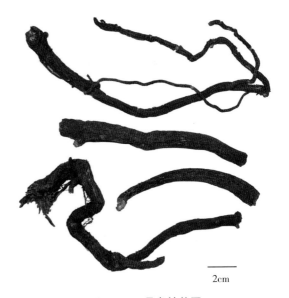

图 23 - 1　丹参性状图

**Figure 23 - 1　Macroscopic characteristics of
Salviae Miltiorrhizae Radix et Rhizoma**

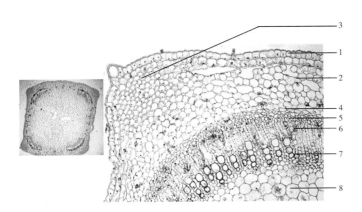

图 23 - 2　薄荷（茎）横切面

**Figure 23 - 2　Transverse section of Menthae
Haplpcalycis Herba（stem）**

1. 表皮细胞（epidermal cells）；2. 皮层（cortex）；

3. 厚角细胞（collenchyma cells）；4. 内皮层（endodermis）；

5. 韧皮部（phloem）；6. 形成层（cambium）；

7. 木质部（xylem）；8. 髓部（pith）

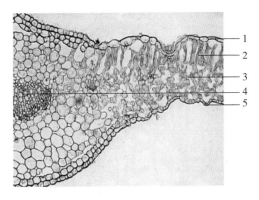

图 23 - 3　薄荷叶横切面

**Figure 23 - 3　Transverse section of Menthae
Haplpcalycis Herba（leaf）**

1. 表皮细胞（epidermal cells）；

2. 栅栏组织（palisade tissue）；

3. 海绵组织（spongy tissue）；

4. 主脉维管束（vascular bundles of main vein）；

5. 下表皮细胞（lower epidermal cells）

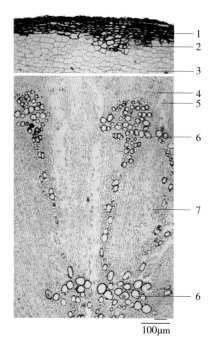

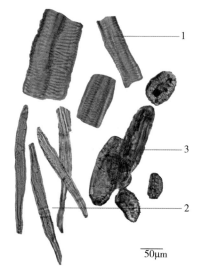

图 23－4　丹参（根）横切面特征图

Figure 23－4　Transverse section of Salviae Miltiorrhizae Radix et Rhizoma

1. 木栓层（cork）；2. 石细胞（sclereid）；3. 皮层（cortex）；

4. 韧皮部（phloem）；5. 形成层（cambium）；

6. 木质部（xylem）；7. 射线（rays）

图 23－5　丹参粉末显微特征图

Figure 23－5　Main powder characteristics of Salviae Miltiorrhizae Radix et Rhizoma

1. 导管（vessels）；2. 木纤维（woody fibres）；

3. 石细胞（sclereid）

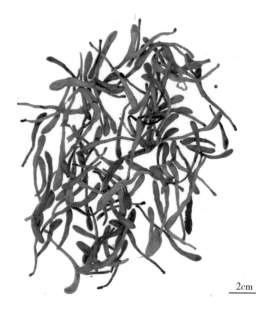

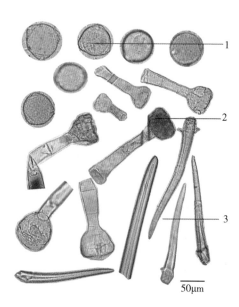

图 24－1　金银花性状图

Figure 24－1　Macroscopic characteristics of Lonicerae Japonicae Flos

图 24－2　金银花粉末显微特征图

Figure 24－2　Main powder characteristics of Lonicerae Japonicae Flos

1. 花粉粒（pollen grains）；2. 腺毛（glandular hairs）；

3. 非腺毛（non－glandular hairs）

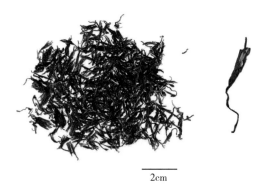

图 25 – 1　红花性状图

Figure 25 – 1　Macroscopic characteristics of Carthami Flos

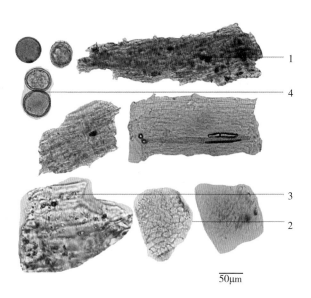

图 26 – 2　西红花粉末显微特征图

Figure 26 – 2　Main powder characteristics of Croci Stigma

1. 表皮细胞（epidermal cells）；

2. 柱头顶端表皮细胞（terminal epidermal cells of stigma）；

3. 草酸钙结晶（crystals of calcium oxalate）；

4. 花粉粒（pollen grains）

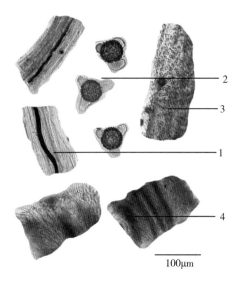

图 25 – 2　红花粉末显微特征图

Figure 25 – 2　Main powder characteristics of Carthami Flos

1. 分泌细胞（secretory cells）；2. 花粉粒（pollen grains）；

3. 花冠碎片（corolla fragments）；4. 柱头碎片（stigma fragments）

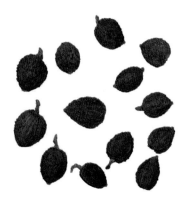

图 27 – 1　砂仁性状图

Figure 27 – 1　Macroscopic characteristics of Amomi Fructus（*Amomum villosum*）

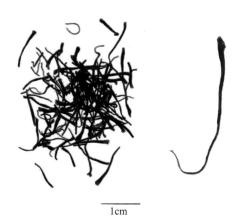

图 26 – 1　西红花性状图

Figure 26 – 1　Macroscopic characteristics of Croci Stigma

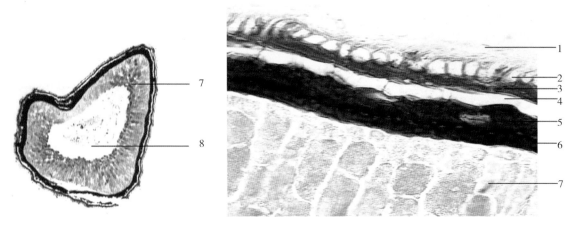

图 27 − 2 阳春砂种子横切面

Figure 27 − 2 Transverse section of Amomi Fructus（seed from *A. villosum*）

1. 假种皮（aril）；2. 种皮表皮细胞（epidermal cells of testa）；3. 下皮细胞（hypodermal cells）；

4. 油细胞（oil cells）；5. 色素层（pigment layer）；

6. 内种皮栅状厚壁细胞（palisade sclerenchymatous cells of endotesta）；

7. 胚乳（endosperm）；8. 胚（embryo）

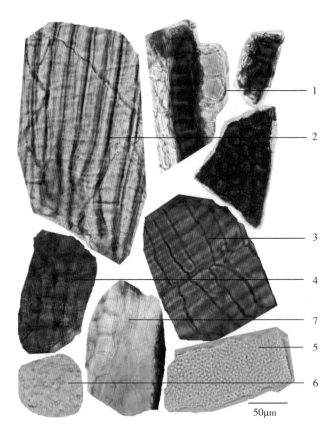

50μm

图 27 − 3 砂仁粉末显微特征图

Figure 27 − 3 Main powder characteristics of Amomi Fructus

1. 内种皮厚壁细胞［sclerenchymatous cells of endotesta（a. 表面观 surface view；b. 断面观 section view）］；

2. 种皮表皮细胞（epidermal cells of testa）；3. 下皮细胞（epidermal cells of testa）；

4. 色素层细胞（pigment layer cells）；5. 外胚乳细胞（perisperm cells）；

6. 内胚乳细胞（endosperm cells）；7. 油细胞（oil cells）

18

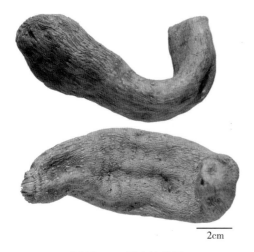

图 28 - 1　天麻性状图

Figure 28 - 1　Macroscopic characteristics of Gastrodiae Rhizoma

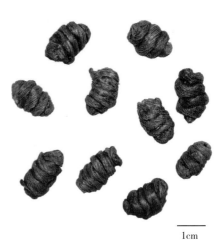

1cm

图 28 - 2　石斛性状图

Figure 28 - 2　Macroscopic characteristics of Dendrobii Calius（*Dendrobium nobile*）

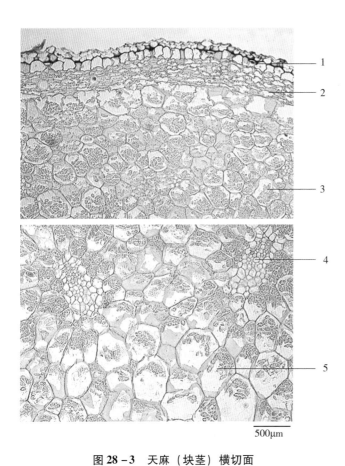

500μm

图 28 - 3　天麻（块茎）横切面

Figure 28 - 3　Transverse section of Gastrodiae Rhizoma

1. 下皮（hypodermis）；2. 皮层（cortex）；3. 中柱（stele）；

4. 维管束（vascular bundles）；5. 髓（pith）

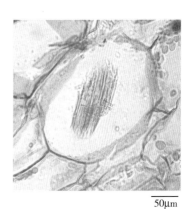

50μm

图 28 - 4　示草酸钙针晶束

Figure 28 - 4　Showing raphides of calcium oxalate

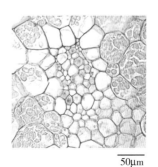

50μm

图 28 - 5　示周韧维管束

Figure 28 - 5　Showing amphicribral vascular bundles

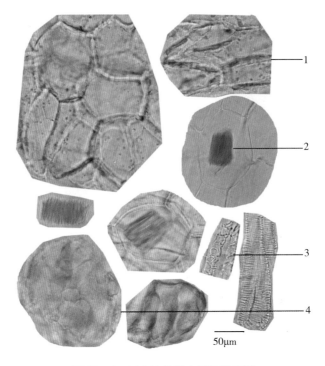

50μm

图 28 - 6 天麻块茎粉末显微特征图

Figure 28 - 6 Main powder characteristics of Gastrodiae Rhizoma

1. 厚壁细胞（sclerenchymatous cells）；2. 草酸钙针晶束（raphides of calcium oxalate）；

3. 含糊化多糖类物的薄壁细胞（parenchymatous cells containing gelatinized polysaccharides）；4. 导管（vessels）

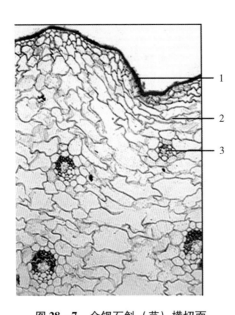

图 28 - 7 金钗石斛（茎）横切面

Figure 28 - 7 Transverse section of Dendrobii Caulis（stem of *D. nobile*）

1. 表皮（epidermis）；2. 薄壁组织（parenchyma）；

3. 维管束（vascular bundles）

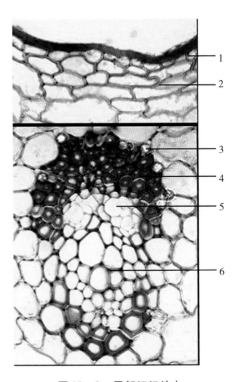

图 28 - 8 局部组织放大

Figure 28 - 8 Magnified partial tissue

1. 表皮（epidermis）；2. 薄壁组织（parenchyma）；

3. 硅质块（siliceous block）；4. 纤维束（fibre bundles）；

5. 韧皮部（phloem）；6. 木质部（xylem）

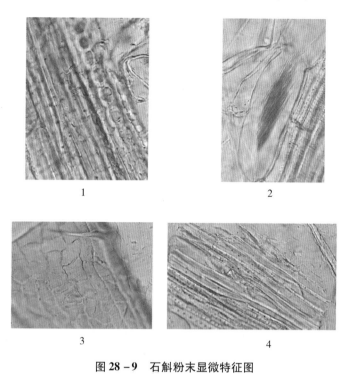

图 28 - 9　石斛粉末显微特征图

Figure 28 - 9　Main powder characteristics of Dendrobii Caulis

1. 束鞘纤维（fibers belong to vessel）；2. 草酸钙针晶（raphides of calcium oxalates）；

3. 表皮细胞（epidermal cells）；4. 木纤维（woody fibres）

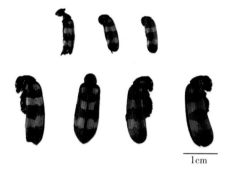

图 29 - 1　斑蝥性状图

Figure 29 - 1　Macroscopic characteristics of Mylabris

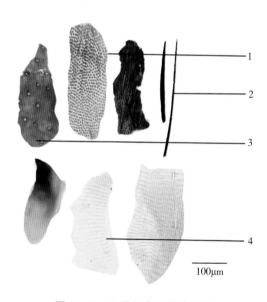

图 29 - 3　斑蝥粉末显微特征图

Figure 29 - 3　Main powder characteristics
of Mylabris

1. 体表碎片（fragments of body walls）；2. 刚毛（setae）；

3. 横纹肌（striped muscle）；4. 鞘翅（elytrum）

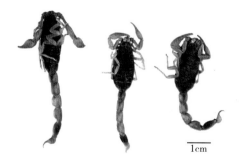

图 29 - 2　全蝎性状图

Figure 29 - 2　Macroscopic characteristics of Scorpio

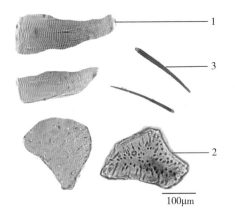

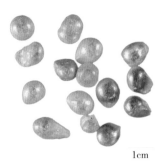

图 29 - 4　全蝎粉末显微特征图

Figure 29 - 4　Main powder characteristics of Scorpio

1. 横纹肌（striped muscle）；2. 体壁碎片（fragments of body walls）；
3. 刚毛（setae）

图 30 - 1　珍珠性状图

**Figure 30 - 1　Macroscopic characteristics
of Margarita**

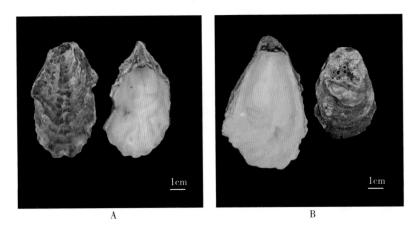

A　　　　　　　　　　　　　B

图 30 - 2　牡蛎性状图

Figure 30 - 2　Macroscopic characteristics of Ostreae Concha

A：大连湾牡蛎壳（*Ostrea talienwhanensis* Crosse）；B：近江牡蛎壳（*Ostrea rivularis* Gould）

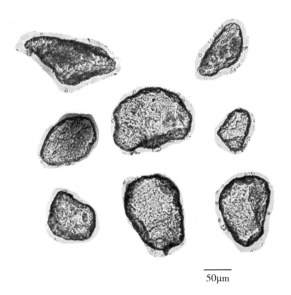

图 30 - 3　珍珠粉末显微特征图

Figure 30 - 3　Main powder characteristics of Margarita

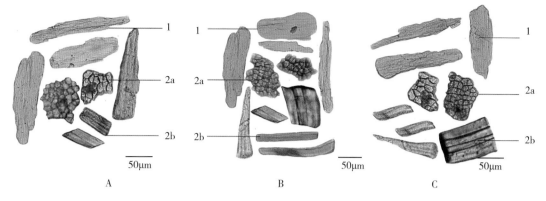

图 30 – 4　牡蛎粉末显微特征图

Figure 30 – 4　Main powder characteristics of Ostreae Concha

A. 长牡蛎（*Ostrea gigas* Thunberg）；B. 大连湾牡蛎（*Ostrea talienwhanensis* Crosse）；C. 近江牡蛎（*Ostrea rivularis* Gould）
1. 珍珠层碎片（nacreous layers pieces）；2a. 棱柱层碎片径向面观（radial view of prismatic layers pieces）；
2b. 棱柱层碎片横断面观（cross section view of prismatic layers pieces）

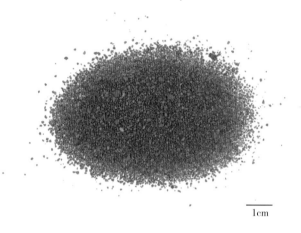

图 31 – 1　朱砂性状图

Figure 31 – 1　Macroscopic characteristics of Cinnabaris

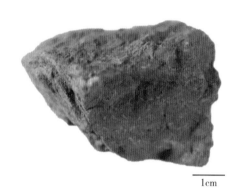

图 31 – 2　雄黄性状图

Figure 31 – 2　Macroscopic characteristics of Realgar